SUCCESS STORIES

"Even after healing from AIP, I had this nagging issue that was balance and dizziness. I had seen a lot of practitioners and no one could get to the bottom of it. I went to see Titus and the information that he gave me was just so valuable and amazing. I began to see improvements in my symptoms in that very first visit. It was very clear that he had all this knowledge that is missing from the autoimmune community"

Mickey Trescott
Best-selling author of The Autoimmune Paleo Cookbook

"I can literally say I've climbed some of the highest mountains in the world because of Dr. Chiu. After only a month working with him, a host of my health problems were solved at lightning speed. I no longer feel the intense pain, headaches, fogginess, or anxiety that I was experiencing when I first went to see Dr. Chiu"

Brandy Parker
Portland, OR

"Dr. Titus has been a lifesaver for me. In 2006, I had a serious traumatic brain injury. Upon getting started with Dr. Chiu, I was immediately comforted by his full engagement to eliminating my headaches. He listens, he educates, and most importantly, he puts you in the driver's seat for your health. For once, I'm actually not losing 2 or 3 entire days per month to migraines. Dr. Titus has unquestionably made this possible for me"

Phil M.
Hayward, CA

"Dr. Chiu is that rare combination of a healer who is both educated, informed, scientific and intuitive. His gift to people's lives is to free up their health, their will to live and their sensibility so that they can go out into this world and be an authentic version of who they are really are!"

Allison Fine
Chicago, IL

"My anxiety, heart palpitations, and face flushing are virtually non-existent. I cannot tell you how amazing it feels to be able to take back my life, my livelihood, my happiness, my personality, my confidence and my motivation. I thank Dr. Chiu for helping me figure out the root of the problems, and truly giving me my life back"

Dr. Jessica Lips
Oakland, CA

"I had been suffering from migraine headaches for three years. After only a few weeks on Dr. Chiu's program, I lost weight, gained energy, was in great spirits, and -- best of all -- completely eliminated the remaining headaches! I credit Dr. Chiu for allowing me to take my life back and can't thank him enough"

Gary H.
Chicago, IL

"I had a treatment to stop my motion sickness and for the first time in my life I could travel- even read- and not feel sick! You truly have changed my life, forever, for the better!"

Suzanne Nash
Chicago, IL

"Since seeing Dr. Chiu, my vertigo has improved substantially, I no longer have headaches every day and I have more energy!"

Mitzi Lorentzen

"I highly recommend Dr. Chiu. I feel like a new person with my brain in balance. The nutritional knowledge I have obtain for my body has helped me to lose weight and keep constant energy levels throughout the day"

Dr. Mandy McManis
Hayward, CA

"Dr. Chiu is the only doctor who was able to see the big picture of my health. I've been all over the country and seen some other amazing doctors, but he was the one who was able to find the missing keys with simple solutions. I trust him with all my health questions now"

Shirin A.
Berkeley, CA

BrainSAVE!

BrainSAVE!

The 6-Week Plan to Heal Your Brain from Concussions, Brain Injuries & Trauma without Drugs or Surgery

DR. TITUS CHIU

ISBN-13: 978-1-7323344-0-3

The Modern Brain
2730 Telegraph Avenue
Berkeley, CA 94705

Book cover design by MKF Cornett / mkfabila.com
Book format by Danielle Holtzer Hawkins
Author photograph by John Dahlgren

This book is dedicated to my Mom and Dad –
who instilled in me from a very young age the value of
hard work, persistence, curiosity, transcendence, faith, and contribution.
Who encouraged me to go out and make a difference in the world.

Without your lifelong love and support,
my healing and this book would never have been possible.

CONTENTS

How to Use this Book

I get it. You're dizzy, you have brain fog, and when you try to read or look at a computer or scroll through your smartphone, your brain and eyeballs feel like they're about to implode. You feel nauseous, your head hurts and you wish you could just get your old self, your old life, and your old brain back.

Having suffered multiple head injuries myself and having worked with thousands of patients over the years, I know what you're going through. That's why I wrote this book.

In it you'll find a collection of the most cutting-edge and natural approaches to healing your brain after a concussion.

This book is jam packed full of information– and I deliberately wrote it this way– because I firmly believe in the power of education to transform healthcare for the millions of people around the world suffering from Post-Concussion Syndrome.

That being said, I've also packed this book to the brim full of practical tips and actions you can take to start healing your brain today. Because it's not just knowledge and understanding alone that will heal your brain. Just as important are the ACTIONS that you will be taking that will lead to your healing and recovery.

And periods of INACTION as you'll also learn. So take your time and be gentle with yourself as you go through these pages.

Part I

In Part I you'll learn WHY your brain isn't working after your concussion and WHAT you can do about it.

You'll learn why the conventional approach to concussion doesn't work.

I'll introduce you to my unique approach to brain healing called Root Cause Neurology.

I'll share with you the TOP 5 BrainSAVE! Neural Networks that are the ROOT CAUSE for your concussion symptoms.

You will also find self-assessment quizzes for each of the five neural networks to help you identify your unique ROOT CAUSE.

And I'll introduce you to BrainSAVE! – the cutting-edge brain healing program I designed to specifically address the ROOT CAUSE for Post-Concussion Syndrome.

Part II

In Part II I'll bust apart a huge MYTH about the brain and introduce you to a scientific breakthrough that will change your life.

Then you'll learn the 12 Biggest Obstacles to Healing from a Concussion.

You'll find another self-assessment quiz to see if one or more of the twelve obstacles are keeping your brain from healing.

Part III

In Part III I'll guide you through my 6-Week BrainSAVE! Plan to Heal Your Brain from Concussions, Brain Injuries & Trauma without Drugs or Surgery.

This is the foundational plan I give to my patients to PRIME their brain cells for the in-person work they'll be doing during their 5-Day BrainSAVE! Recovery Program at my integrative brain wellness center. You'll learn:

- The Top 5 BrainSAVE! Supplements for concussion
- What foods to eat and to avoid to speed up the healing process
- The secret recipe for my BrainSAVE! Keto Shake

- The 7 Foundational BrainSAVE! Exercises to rebuild your brain
- Key BrainSAVE! Lifestyle Strategies
- And much, much more

It's a very comprehensive yet doable plan that will get you started on your road to recovery.

An important note:

BrainSAVE! is for people who have been struggling with the symptoms of Post-Concussion Syndrome months or even years after their initial injury. It is *not* intended for acute traumatic brain injury patients. If you haven't already, be sure to get checked by your doctor to rule out any serious life-threatening injuries before taking on any of the recommendations found in this book.

One final suggestion for those of you who find it difficult to read for very long because of your concussion:

Although the information in Parts I and II is very important so you can understand WHY your brain isn't working, feel free to skip ahead and go directly to the 6-Week BrainSAVE! Plan found in Part III of this book. I won't be offended. My goal in writing BrainSAVE! is for you to get your brain, your health and your life back as quickly as possible.

Within a few weeks on the plan, you should be feeling better. At that point, I encourage you to go back and read Parts I and II to learn WHY your brain isn't working and the science behind HOW the recommendations in the 6-Week Plan actually work.

This stuff is not magic– it's science. The cutting-edge of neuroscience, systems biology and concussion care to be precise. But I do believe that looking at the world magically, and being open to what is possible will ALWAYS contribute to the healing process.

To Your Total Health,

Dr. Titus Chiu, MS, DC, DACNB

Functional Neurologist

www.DrTitusChiu.com

PART I

Why Isn't My Brain Working After My Concussion?

CHAPTER 1

Hope for Healing

S O YOU SMASHED YOUR HEAD and injured your brain.

And since then your life has drastically changed and taken a wrong turn for the worst. You're having brain fog, headaches, dizziness, fatigue, light and sound sensitivity. You startle easily, and feel scattered, forgetful and moody. You can't sleep at night even though you're so exhausted and tired during the day– and when you are able to get some sleep, its fitful and you don't feel at all rested or refreshed when you wake up.

What was second nature to you before your concussion now takes you an eternity to finish, if you're able to finish at all.

It's scary. And frustrating. You don't feel like your old self anymore. Physically, mentally and emotionally.

Why isn't your brain healing after your concussion? Will it heal? Can it heal?? Are there things that you can be doing to get better? Or do you have to just accept your fate?

You feel so confused, scared and alone in all of this. Your loved ones are trying to be there for you, but they too are anxious, concerned, confused, and can't quite fully understand what you're going through.

Because on the surface, you look well enough. There isn't too much physical evidence of your injury– your eyeballs aren't falling out of their sockets. And if you have scars they may not even be that notice-able. Even if they are, the external signs pale in comparison with what you're struggling internally with on a daily basis.

And to make matters worse, you've been to doctor after doctor and specialist after specialist and they don't have anything for you besides some medications to numb your symptoms or generic advice like "get some rest" or "wear sunglasses and take some aspirin".

Or even worse, they completely write you off and tell you that it's all in your head.

Well– I'm here to tell you that yes, it IS all in your head. But not in the way they meant it.

The reason why you're still suffering after your concussion is most definitely caused by a problem in your head. More specifically, imbalances in key areas of your brain known as neural networks– which are IN YOUR HEAD. Encased in the hard bones of your skull.

Post-concussion syndrome is a very real, neurobiological problem deeply rooted in several KEY NEURAL NETWORKS that make up your brain.

And with that radical understanding, treatment and recovery is completely within your reach.

Healing is possible.

My Mission

As a Functional Medicine doctor that specializes in neurology and post-concussion syndrome, I've worked with thousands of patients suffering from complex brain disorders– concussion, traumatic brain injury, anxiety, depression, chronic brain fog, early Alzheimer's and dementia– the list goes on and on.

Whether they were gold medal Olympic athletes, top hockey and soccer players, professional mixed martial artists– or stay at home moms, graduate students, business executives, doctors, lawyers, and entrepreneurs– they all had one thing in common. A brain ravaged by the damaging effects of Post-Concussion Syndrome.

And every single day I see the impact that it has not only on my patients, but also the massive ripple effects it has on their family, friends and loved ones.

It's so sad to see.

I've also witnessed remarkable stories of healing and recovery as well– from relief from the symptoms of post-concussion syndrome, to the reversal of dementia and Alzheimer's, to a lifetime of anxiety being alleviated in just a few months– all without the use of drugs or surgery.

That's why I'm on a mission to share this message of hope– and to transform healthcare for the millions of people around the world suffering from Post-Concussion Syndrome.

I had the recent honor of being featured in Dr. Mark Hyman's groundbreaking Broken Brain documentary. I talked about how it was completely possible to slow, stop and even reverse serious brain disorders. That film was literally watched by millions of people around the world and I couldn't have been happier. I'm determined to get this message of hope and healing out to everyone needing to hear it.

My passion and determination not only come from my experiences as a doctor in the trenches of care, but also from my own healing journey with natural medicine...

My Story

Throughout my career as a professor and Functional Neurologist– for over a decade, I ran a private practice in Chicago, co-founded KOBA– a Functional Medicine Center in Berkeley, California that specializes in brain health and autoimmunity, and traveled all over the world teaching clinical neurology to thousands of students and doctors.

But before I was a professor and doctor and able to teach and serve others– I struggled with many chronic health issues myself– although at the time I didn't attribute them to my own broken brain.

I just resigned myself to the belief that that was just the way I was– that being, unmotivated, tired all the time, brain foggy and constantly getting sick was normal. Little did I know that all my symptoms that I had identified with as "Titus" wasn't who I was but was a result of a brain out of balance.

The breaking point was when I got in a horrible car accident that nearly cost me my life. I was on my way to work one day when I was struck by a car. I was thrown ten feet through the air from my scooter, came crashing down to the ground– broke three ribs, dislocated my shoulder, and bloodied up my face and body.

The impact was so strong that when I finally got my bearings, I noticed that my helmet had come off, even though it had been tightly fastened to my head. Thank God I was wearing a helmet, or I would not be alive today writing this book for you.

Although I survived, I was left in chronic pain and unable to do all the things that I loved. I tried everything– conventional medicine, physical therapy, pain killers– but nothing worked. It wasn't until I discovered natural medicine that I began to address the root cause for all my symptoms and I began to heal. And one of the darkest times in my life turned out to be a blessing in disguise. I had found my life's calling.

It was at that turning point that I decided to dedicate my life to learning as much as I could about the brain and Functional Medicine. I went back to school and completed a 3-year post-doc in Functional Neurology, got my masters in nutrition, became licensed as a chiropractor, got certified in acupuncture and graduated from the Institute for Functional Medicine's flagship AFMCP program.

Along the way, I also attended thousands of hours of continuing education courses and conferences, read hundreds of books and research articles– anything that I could get my hands on. I dove deep– drinking from the vast oceans of knowledge passed down to us from ancient Eastern practices to the latest breakthroughs in brain science, nutrition and Functional Medicine.

And after many years of formal education and learning from the masters of neurology and Functional Medicine– and after thousands of hours synthesizing all this information and experience, I began to identify patterns and fundamental principles. And I found myself flying all over the world, teaching other doctors my unique blend of neurology, nutrition and Functional Medicine that I now call Root Cause Neurology.

A Dream Come True

I had the honor of giving a lecture on the latest breakthroughs in concussion care at the Institute for Functional Medicine's 2017 Annual International Conference on the Brain. It was a dream come true. Three of my deepest passions came together at that conference: teaching, Functional Medicine and the Brain.

And what a conference it was! Over 1400 doctors, chiropractors, naturopaths, acupuncturists, nutritionists, NYT bestselling authors, thought leaders and philanthropists flew in from around the globe for this most worthy of causes: to revolutionize and transform healthcare for the over 1 billion people around the globe suffering from brain disorders. I was so honored to share the stage with other thought leaders and giants in the world of neurology and Functional Medicine: Dr. David Perlmutter, Dr. Dale Bredesen, Dr. Mark Hyman, Dr. Norman Doidge, Dr. Michael Merzenich, Dr. Terry Wahls, Dr. Datis Kharrazian and many more.

What you hold in your hands right now are the key points of that talk, as well as the culmination of years of study, research, treating patients, teaching doctors and healing my own brain.

It contains solutions for your post-concussion symptoms that have worked for me and the countless patients I've worked with over the years.

Welcome to BrainSAVE!

CHAPTER 2

Post-Concussion Syndrome

A Silent, Global Epidemic

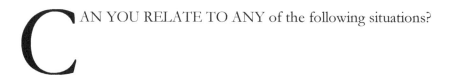

C AN YOU RELATE TO ANY of the following situations?

- Frustrated that you can't do the things you used to be able to do? And when you do simple tasks, it takes twice as long to do them and it wipes you out and you feel completely frazzled or exhausted?
- Worried that you'll lose your job because you can't think clearly anymore or are unfocused and forgetful?
- Anxious if you'll ever get better?

- Plagued with anxiety that never existed, at least to this level prior to your head injury?
- Annoyed with the lack of answers and clarity about what's actually going on?
- Upset at being written off by doctors?
- Sad that you don't have the energy or focus to be present with your friends, family or kids?
- Alone because no one seems to understand what you're going through?
- Hopeless?

If so, you can take comfort in the fact that you are not alone. Almost all of the patients I've seen have felt the way you do and the way I did– and struggled with the same symptoms that you are struggling with. How do I know? Because they told me! These are all very common symptoms associated with Post-Concussion Syndrome– a very real brain disorder that has been profoundly unaddressed by conventional medicine.

The Spectrum of Traumatic Brain Injury

At this point you're probably wondering– what exactly is Post-Concussion Syndrome? Post-Concussion Syndrome or PCS for short– is a very real medical condition that falls under a spectrum of brain disorders known as traumatic brain injuries or TBI.

Concussion

It starts with a concussion, or a blow to your head. That blow to your head is what is known as a mild traumatic brain injury– a head injury with a temporary loss of brain function. It's the most common form of TBI.

The scary thing is, you don't even need to experience an actual blow to the head to have had a concussion. I've seen so many patients suffering from the symptoms of PCS and claim that they never had a head injury or concussion. Upon further investigation though I find out that they were in a big car accident and/or suffered whiplash– but didn't actually hit their head.

Or they were tossed around on a rollercoaster and jarred their head– but again no actual blow to the head *or loss of consciousness*. But after that jarring is when all of their symptoms began.

And that's the thing– concussions don't have to involve a loss of consciousness or even a blow to the head. That's why they're such a silent and deadly epidemic.

Post-Concussion Syndrome

So the blow to the head or even a strong jolt that shakes your brain up, is what's called a concussion. Post-Concussion Syndrome on the other hand is the set of *symptoms* that lingers for weeks, months or even years after the initial concussion. Post-Concussion Syndrome is not the head injury itself– but rather refers to the set of *symptoms* that may accompany concussion. Symptoms of Post-Concussion Syndrome can be divided into physical, mental and emotional.

PHYSICAL SYMPTOMS:	MENTAL SYMPTOMS	EMOTIONAL SYMPTOMS
• Headaches • Dizziness • Insomnia • Fuzzy or blurry vision • Sensitivity to light or sound • Balance problems • Physical fatigue	• Brain fog • Hard time thinking clearly • Slowed reaction time • Problems with concentration • Difficulty remembering new information • Feeling scatter-brained • Mental fatigue	• Irritability • Sadness • More emotional • Nervousness • Anxiety • Depression

Any of these ring a bell? These are all typical symptoms of a concussion– and most people recover quickly and completely from them. But if your symptoms have lasted for more than two months after your head injury then you may very well be suffering from Post-Concussion Syndrome.

Chronic Traumatic Encephalopathy

And finally, there's chronic traumatic encephalopathy or CTE. This is the end game– where the initial concussion (or concussions) turns into a deadly neurodegenerative process that can be only diagnosed after death, when the brain is analyzed for signs of shrinkage and toxic plaques.

The brains of people with CTE look very similar to the brains of people with Alzheimer's disease. One of the major differences is that while Alzheimer's disease usually affects people in their 60s or 70s, evidence for chronic traumatic encephalopathy has been found in people as young as 17 years old![1]

The good news is that not everyone that has a concussion develops CTE, but it's a lot more common than once suspected.

The spectrum of Concussion, Post-Concussion Syndrome and Chronic Traumatic Encephalopathy truly is a silent, global epidemic.

- TBI accounts for approximately 10 million deaths and/or hospitalizations annually in the world and approximately 1.5

million annual emergency room visits and hospitalizations in the US.

- In the United States alone, it's responsible for 30% of all injury-related deaths. In 2010, 2.5 million people suffered a traumatic brain injury.

- Every day, 153 people in the United States alone dies from injuries that include traumatic brain injury.

- TBI results in $330,827 of average lifetime costs associated with disability and lost productivity and greatly outweighs the $65,504 estimated costs for initial medical care and rehab.

- About 75% of TBIs that occur each year are concussions or other forms of mild TBI, but even so-called mild TBI usually lead to enduring cognitive deficits.

- Half of all traumatic deaths in the US are due to brain injury and the majority of head injuries are considered mild and patients often never receive medical treatment.[2]

What ends up happening to all these patients who never received treatment? We suffer in silence while our lives fall apart all around us. And even when we do seek out care, we find that there really isn't much out there.

To make matters even worse, untreated concussions **significantly increase the risk for serious neurological and/or psychiatric conditions**[3] such as dementia[4], Alzheimer's disease[5], Parkinson's disease[6], multiple sclerosis[7], anxiety and depression[8]. I've even worked with many patients with Hashimoto's– an autoimmune disease impacting the thyroid– that they developed after sustaining a concussion!

IMPORTANT SIDE NOTE

This is due to the fact that brain injuries can cause leaky gut[9]– which is one of three factors needed to trigger autoimmunity[10]. I was able to help them reverse their Hashimoto's by healing both their gut *and* their brains.

CHAPTER 3

The Problem with the Standard of Care

S O WHY ARE THERE SO many people still suffering from the symptoms of concussion?

I see three main reasons for this:

1. **There just aren't enough doctors trained in the latest concussion diagnosis and treatment protocols. Period.**

Why else would there be so many people still suffering from concussion? And why else would you still be searching for answers? I can't tell you how many patients I've spoken to who have told me that they had been seen by the top concussion specialists in the world– and all the advice they were given was to get some rest or take some aspirin!

That's one of the main reasons why I decided to write this book– to give you access to cutting-edge protocols so you can take control of your brain health today.

2. There is typically a 20-year lag between scientific discoveries and the practical application of treatments based on those discoveries.

Although the scientific breakthroughs that form the basis of Brain-SAVE! were discovered by scientists and researchers many years ago, they still haven't been translated into standard treatments you'd find at a visit to your doctor's office. I want to shorten that gap and get this cutting-edge information into your hands TODAY and give you some safe and powerful tools and actions that you can take so you can begin the healing process NOW.

Not twenty years from now– after you've already suffered a lifetime of crippling anxiety, brain fog and depression. Or you've already developed Alzheimer's, chronic traumatic encephalopathy or any one of the serious neurological disorders that can be triggered as a result of untreated concussions.

I've taken the best, safest, most natural therapies that eastern and western medicine have to offer, combined them and laid them out for you in Part III of this book.

BrainSAVE! will show you what the ROOT CAUSES are for your post-concussion symptoms, and how to address them using safe, natural, clinically-proven, science-based strategies, without the use of drugs riddled with unwanted side-effects or invasive surgeries.

I want you to be able to live a life of abundance, and joy, and peace, and serenity and focus and meaning– and to do all the things that you love doing, according to your values and the things that are most important to you.

3. The third and final reason is that traditional neurology and conventional medicine solely focuses on the diagnosis, and treatment is geared towards suppressing the symptoms associated with that diagnosis.

What's wrong with that approach, you ask?

Well, all a diagnosis is, is a fancy label for a collection of different SYMPTOMS. A diagnosis doesn't tell you WHY you're still suffering from your concussion or why your brain isn't working. It just puts a label on it.

And usually the "treatments" involve just a temporary masking of symptoms– kind of like putting a Band-Aid on a dam that's about to burst.

I understand that while receiving a diagnosis after struggling with the fear and uncertainty of some strange neurological disorder may give you some peace of mind. Or getting temporary relief from your pain and headaches is better than no relief at all. But I want even more for you.

I want us to dive deeper to find out WHY you're still struggling after your concussion so you can know WHAT to do to have long-term relief from your symptoms. So more important than any label or diagnosis is understanding the ROOT CAUSE for your chronic concussion symptoms.

Symptoms vs Roots

Symptoms are like the leaves on a tree. If your tree has a bunch of leaves that are brown or shriveled up and you want your tree looking healthy and vibrant again you have several options. One option is to go out and buy some paint and paint the leaves a pretty gold or green or red color. It might look nice at first, but since the cause isn't being addressed the leaves continue to get sicker and sicker and eventually fall off and die. The solution is temporary and cosmetic.

Another option is to figure out why the leaves are sick to begin with. Most of the time it's because there are underlying imbalances buried deep underground and lurking in the roots of the tree, hidden from plain sight. It's at this level we need to focus our energy and attention if you want solid and long-lasting results.

The same goes for your brain. When you experience things like headaches, fatigue, brain fog, memory problems or irritability – it's just your body's way of telling you that there's something wrong. That there's an underlying imbalance – a ROOT CAUSE – somewhere in your nervous system that needs care and attention.

We can try to mask the symptom with pain killers or medications but in addition to unwanted side effects my biggest problem with this approach is it doesn't address the ROOT CAUSE for your symptoms. And in the long run, many of the medications end up causing more harm than the initial health issue you were trying to fix!

Masking the symptoms with medications is like removing the light bulb to the "check engine" signal in your car. Or taking out the battery to the fire alarm going off in your house. And in the long run can actually cause more harm than good. Out of sight out of mind– for now. Until your car completely breaks down or your house burns down.

I don't want to come off sounding completely negative about the conventional medical system. If I was ever in another major car accident and suffered serious injuries, I would definitely want to be sent to the emergency room and be seen by conventional doctors. I'd want to make sure that my injuries weren't life threatening and if they were, to have any surgeries or procedures done that would be needed to save my life.

Because what the conventional medical system excels at is handling life-threatening emergency situations like major car accidents, or acute traumatic brain injuries and bleeds.

But when it comes to the care and management of chronic diseases like Post-Concussion Syndrome and Chronic Traumatic Encephalopathy, we need a completely different approach all together.

We need ROOT CAUSE NEUROLOGY™.

CHAPTER 4

Root Cause Neurology

A T MY INTEGRATIVE NEUROLOGY CENTER, I practice what I call Root Cause Neurology™. I've taken the best of what Eastern and Western medicine have to offer– by combining the art of traditional healing with the latest breakthroughs in neuroscience, systems biology and genomic medicine.

Root Cause Neurology™ forms the basis for both the 5-Day in-office BrainSAVE! Recovery Program, as well as the 6-Week Brain-SAVE! Plan found in Part III of this book.

It's a simple 3-step process that I've developed and refined over the years:

Step 1: Identify the ROOT CAUSE

Step 2: Treat the ROOT CAUSE

Step 3: Remove the OBSTACLES

Using this investigative approach to neurology, I've successfully helped thousands of patients suffering from complex, chronic neurological conditions get their lives back. I even used this approach to fix my own broken brain.

So the first step that's needed to heal from your concussion is to identify the root cause for your post-concussion symptoms.

And the ROOT CAUSE for Post-Concussion Syndrome is ALL IN YOUR HEAD.

CHAPTER 5

Healer Heal Thyself

AFTER DISCOVERING NEUROLOGY AND Functional Medicine it seemed like life for me was so picturesque and ideal. I had a beautiful and supportive wife, ran a busy and successful integrative neurology practice, and was being flown all over the world to speak at conferences to teach other doctors about neurology, nutrition and lifestyle medicine. It was like a dream come true.

On the surface.

But underneath it all, I was struggling. Sure– I had overcome a lot of my old health issues by adopting many of the things that I learned in school and seminars and books– I changed my diet, took supplements, got regular massages and chiropractic care– and through all that I had tons of motivation, had a lot of energy, mental clarity, my skin issues cleared up and I rarely got sick anymore. But even as these chronic health issues began to disappear, other deeper, darker mental health issues slowly started to emerge–depression, anger, excessive worry, paranoia. And while my outer professional life was thriving, my inner personal world was falling apart at the seams.

During this time, I continued to attend hundreds of hours of seminars, researching and learning about the latest advances in neurology, nutrition, Functional Medicine, and concussion care. And I continued to experiment on myself and apply everything that I learned in those seminars to my own life. I got even stricter and more disciplined with my diet– really getting clear on the impact certain foods had on me and my mood. I experimented with cutting-edge healing technologies. I upped my dosage of supplements and I started a daily meditation practice and did more yoga.

And guess what? A lot of those deeper, darker health issues that I had– *that I didn't even realize or acknowledge*– began to resolve.

When I looked back on all of it I was like, "Oh my God," everything that I experimented with that had worked for me, were the same brain healing protocols that I'd been prescribing to my patients with Post-Concussion Syndrome!

And looking back I also realized I had never struggled with any of these darker, psychological symptoms growing up. I was a happy child that came from a great and loving family– I wasn't angry, I wasn't irritable, I didn't excessively worry about things and I definitely didn't suffer from paranoia. These symptoms were completely new to me.

"What was happening to me?", I thought to myself. So I did an in-depth analysis *into my own history*, just like I had done for all my patients.

And it dawned on me.

Many of these deeper, darker mental health issues that I had been silently struggling with had started *after* that fateful car accident so many years ago. But because they had gotten worse slowly over time, *I wasn't even aware that they were there.*

Here I was, Dr. Titus Chiu– a Functional Neurologist specializing in concussion, whose personal life was being torn apart because of a brain imbalance *caused by a concussion*. Like a slow growing tumor, it was taking over my life without me even realizing it.

And it wasn't until I learned how to rebuild my own brain and live in alignment with my higher self that I finally got my life back and I began to heal on an even deeper level.

And in order for you to heal there are three key concepts that you are going to have to accept.

KEY CONCEPT #1: Your Brain CAN Heal

To heal your brain you need to accept this fact– your brain *can* and *will* heal when the ROOT CAUSE is identified, you're given the right treatment for your unique neurology, genetics and brain chemistry, and when the biggest obstacles to your healing are removed. This is Root Cause Neurology™.

KEY CONCEPT #2: It's ALL IN YOUR HEAD

The ROOT CAUSE for your post-concussion symptoms is all in your head– located in key neural networks that make up your brain and create your experience of life.

KEY CONCEPT #3: It's All Connected

Although the ROOT CAUSE for Post-Concussion Syndrome is in your head, some of the major obstacles keeping your brain from healing aren't. Rather, they're located in the other systems of your body. And since your brain is intimately connected to your body– digestive, immune, hormonal, detoxification, and mitochondrial imbalances can all be major roadblocks to recovery from Post-Concussion Syndrome.

The Doctor's Doctor

I never planned on becoming a Post-Concussion Syndrome specialist. My original focus was working with patients dealing with more general health issues like chronic fatigue and chronic pain and other chronic conditions.

Because of my deep passion and drive to learn as much as I could about health and the healing arts– I was getting some pretty good results even as a young doctor right out of school.

In addition, I was teaching a post-doctorate program in clinical neurology for a very prestigious neurology institute, and traveling all over the world training other doctors in neurology.

For these reasons I ended up getting a lot of referrals from my colleagues as well as other doctors who had been in practice much longer than I had been. Many of these doctors themselves became patients of mine– so I could help them resolve their own chronic health issues.

I became known in my professional circles as "the Doctor's Doctor".

So over the years I had the opportunity to work with thousands of patients with complex health issues– and for the most part I was getting great results with them. But during this time I also saw a group of patients that weren't responding to my care, no matter what I tried.

I was stumped.

So I dug deeper and discovered that the common denominator for many of them was a history of one or more traumatic brain injuries.

When I realized that– I did what I was born to do. I went deep– deep into the neuroscience of concussion– and I attended even more seminars specifically on concussion, and read scientific article after scientific article, researching the latest concussion treatment protocols. And guess what? When I applied what I'd learned with these patients many of them finally started to get better.

Because of this I have had the unique opportunity to work with countless people over the years struggling with Post-Concussion Syndrome, helping them get their lives back.

And since then I've found even more patterns– connecting the dots between their post-concussion symptoms, the specific brain regions affected, and matching that with the right treatment.

And so patients fly in from all over the world to see me, often after seeing many other doctors and healthcare providers– both within conventional and alternative medicine. They know that something is wrong, even though most if not all of their tests come back normal.

But they've given up on the conventional medical approach of more and more medications and truly want to figure it out once and for all.

The people who I love working with and that get the most out of my brain healing programs come with a willingness to learn and a desire to explore and understand the ROOT CAUSE for their neurological symptoms.

And the people that recover the quickest are the ones that do the work, are committed to the healing process, and follow through with the recommendations that I personalize for them, after identifying the ROOT CAUSE for their symptoms.

So what is the ROOT CAUSE for Post-Concussion Syndrome?

CHAPTER 6

It's All in Your Head

ALL THE ANNOYING SYMPTOMS OF Post-Concussion Syndrome such as brain fog, fatigue, headaches, dizziness, balance problems, forgetfulness, memory problems, irritability, light and sound sensitivity, distractibility, poor focus and concentration, insomnia, anxiety, and depression– are caused by imbalances in **KEY NEURAL NETWORKS** that make up your brain. They determine whether you feel happy or sad, focused or scattered, healthy or in pain.

What the heck are NEURAL NETWORKS?

Ahhhh, your amazing human brain. It allows you to think, to feel, to move, to create, to learn, to grow– and to love. You're able to experience all of that because of the communication that's happening between your brain cells, brain regions and neural networks.

Cells, Regions and Neural Networks

Your itty bitty little brain cell– where it all begins. But even though the diameter of each of your brain cells is about the width of a piece of dust, your nervous system contains over 100 billion brain cells. In fact, you have more brain cells sitting in between your two ears than there are stars in the galaxy!

And each brain cell connects with over 10,000 other brain cells. Brain cells that live close to one another form what are known as brain regions. And each brain region has its own unique function.

But the star of the show are your neural networks. Because it's through activation and deactivation patterns of these neural networks that give you your experience of the world within you and around you.

Your neural networks are involved with and create virtually every experience you have as a human being. There are neural networks for falling in love, for enjoying music, for dancing, for gratitude and for compassion. All the truly wonderful things in life.

When they're working.

When they're not, you'll end up experiencing all of the horrible symptoms of concussion that you've been struggling with. When they become damaged, as they do after a head injury, they can become the source for much of your suffering.

Weak, broken, and imbalanced neural networks are the ROOT CAUSE for all of your post-concussion symptoms.

In order to get you back on the road to recovery, it is CRITICAL that you identify which of your neural networks have been damaged so that the appropriate treatment can be rendered and you can get your brain and your life back.

KAREN'S STORY

Karen flew in to see me from Hawaii after she saw me give a talk at an international conference on anxiety.

She had been struggling with chronic fatigue for several years. One day, while she was out of town traveling for work, she passed out and ended up in the hospital. Earlier that day, she was feeling dizzier than usual but never thought she would be rushed to the ER.

As I went deeper into her history, I discovered that she had suffered a concussion a month before the incident. She had slipped on some ice, hit the back of her head and briefly lost consciousness. She was so busy at the time having just graduated from law school and so didn't seek any care.

In addition to her chronic fatigue she also reported brain fog, mental disorganization and distractibility, headaches, dizziness, motion sickness, light and sound sensitivity, forgetfulness and insomnia.

Upon further questioning I discovered that in addition to her recent concussion, she had suffered at least four to five other concussions that she described as "pretty bad". While playing soccer in college, she suffered a concussion so severe that she had to quit the team. She suffered another serious head injury when she was in a car accident. She felt nauseous afterwards and went to the hospital to get checked out but as is usually the case with concussion, all the tests came back "normal".

Since then her memory had been progressively getting worse, she was experiencing massive brain fog and found it really difficult to focus at work. The thing that concerned her the most though was her severe anxiety. She told me that she was never really anxious before her most recent head injury, and that the anxiety was really impacting her ability as a lawyer. She described it as a "panicked feeling" in the "pit of her gut".

She had seen many doctors and tried everything they recommended but nothing was able to give her any real lasting solutions.

What was going on with Karen? And why did all her tests come back "normal"?

After taking a comprehensive and in-depth look at her history, I performed an advanced neurological exam. I looked at how her eyes moved, I checked her balance, I had her move her fingers and arms to see how coordinated and fast her movements were, I shined a light in her eyes to look at how her pupils contracted, I checked her reflexes and muscle strength.

I ran many different neurological tests on her, some similar to the ones that the previous doctors she saw had run that had come up "normal".

But the main difference was how I interpreted the findings of the exam. Looking very intently, I could see that her eyes would move quickly to the right, but slower to the left. I also noticed that she had an easier time balancing on her right foot versus her left. And that when she tapped her fingers together, she was a lot slower with her left hand versus her right.

What did it all mean?

Although Karen's findings were extremely subtle, such that her previous doctors didn't recognize them and declared them as "normal", *I knew they were the keys to cracking her case.* I've observed these subtle findings with every single one of the patients I've worked with who has had a concussion. And their subtle findings were the keys to solving their cases as well.

You see, the subtle changes in how her eyes moved, or her difficulty balancing or moving her fingers and arms didn't just mean that her eyes, fingers and legs were "weak". They were the *critical clues* as to which of her NEURAL NETWORKS were weak, broken and imbalanced. Concrete, measurable, objective findings pointing to the underlying ROOT CAUSE for all her symptoms.

But because the findings aren't easily detectable to an untrained eye that's not taught to look for these subtleties, they are so often missed. Which is why so many patients with Post-Concussion Syndrome fall through the cracks of conventional medicine.

I knew this, so I had my team videotape the neurological evaluation so I could play it back for her– and point out the subtleties for her to see and understand. Because I knew it was that important– based on the thousands of patients I've seen over the years, each of them presenting with different yet subtle findings.

They were windows into her broken neural networks.

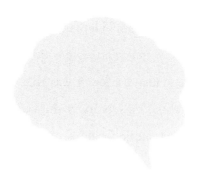

CHAPTER 7

The Top 5 BrainSAVE! Neural Networks

THERE ARE LITERALLY HUNDREDS OF different brain regions and neural networks that can get injured in a concussion. That's why it's IMPERATIVE to get an advanced neurological evaluation by a Functional Neurology specialist trained in Post-Concussion Syndrome– so they can tease apart which specific neural networks are at the root cause for YOUR symptoms (see Brain-Boosting Resources at the end of this book).

That being said, I'd like to introduce you to the **TOP 5 Brain-SAVE! Neural Networks.** These are the five most commonly injured neural networks that I've seen in my patients with Post-Concussion

Syndrome. As you read about the Top 5 BrainSAVE! Neural Net-works, check to see if you can relate to any of the listed symptoms.

This will help you identify YOUR unique BrainSAVE! imbalances, which just might be the ROOT CAUSE for all your post-concussion symptoms.

NOTE

As you're learning about the different neural networks, feel free to begin scoring each of them (see instructions below). At the end of this section, you'll be taking your total scores so you can iden-tify your unique BrainSAVE! imbalances to find out what you can do about them.

NEURAL NETWORK #1: Prefrontal Cortex

Where it's at:

Your Prefrontal Cortex is one of the four lobes that make up your brain. It sits directly behind your forehead– so it's very susceptible to damage after a concussion.

What it does:

Your Prefrontal Cortex is part of several key neural networks whose main jobs are to keep you focused, help you concentrate, organize your thoughts, plan for the future, calm your emotions and prevent you from acting inappropriately.

Clues that something's wrong:

Damage to your Prefrontal Cortex is at the ROOT CAUSE for the following Post-Concussion Syndrome symptoms:

Scoring:

Place a 0, 1, 2 or 3 next to each symptom to grade its severity.

0 = none, 1 = mild, 2 = moderate and 3 = severe

Brain Fog	
Depression	
Distractibility	
Problems with focus and concentration	
Short term memory issues	
Addictions	
Hypersexuality	
Impulsivity	
Always running late to appointments	
Lack of motivation	
TOTAL SCORE	

NEURAL NETWORK #2: Temporal Lobe

Where it's at:

Your Temporal Lobe is another of the four major lobes that make up your brain. It sits above your ears and behind your temples and is also very susceptible to injury after a concussion.

What it does:

The Temporal Lobe is part of a neural network whose main job is to consolidate your experiences for long-term memory storage. It's also important for regulating your mood, stress management, sound processing, and understanding what you read and hear.

Clues that something's wrong:

Trauma to your temporal lobe can lead to the following Post-Concussion Syndrome symptoms:

Scoring:

Place a 0, 1, 2 or 3 next to each symptom to grade its severity.

0 = none, 1 = mild, 2 = moderate and 3 = severe

Stress	
Anger	
Irritability	
Paranoia	
Feeling spaced out	
Changes in your hearing	
Poor language comprehension	
Memory impairment	
Hearing or smelling things that aren't there	
Seizures	
TOTAL SCORE	

NEURAL NETWORK #3: Cerebellum

Where it's at:

Although your cerebellum is pretty small when compared to the rest of your brain (it only makes up 10% of its total weight), it contains more cells than the rest of your brain combined. It sits underneath the back part of your brain and is also very susceptible to trauma after a concussion.

What it does:

Although classically involved with control of your muscles and movements, recent research has implicated the cerebellum playing an important role in immune health and emotional well-being.

Clues that something's wrong:

Injury to the cerebellum can lead to the following Post-Concussion Syndrome symptoms:

Scoring:

Place a 0, 1, 2 or 3 next to each symptom to grade its severity.

0 = none, 1 = mild, 2 = moderate and 3 = severe

Balance problems	
Clumsiness	
Tremors	
Chronic neck and back pain	
Headaches and dizziness	
Problems smoothly coordinating your movements together	
Difficulty connecting your thoughts	
Slurred speech	
Blurred vision	
Chronic ankle or shoulder sprains	
TOTAL SCORE	

<u>NEURAL NETWORK #4</u>: Brainstem

Where it's at:

This essential part of your nervous system sits between your brain and spinal cord and can be broken up into three main regions– top, middle and bottom.

What it does:

Your brainstem is a major hub for key neural networks that orchestrate life-sustaining vital functions such as your heart beat, breathing and digestion, and sleep/wake cycles.

The top part of your brainstem– also known as the midbrain, sets your sleep/wake cycle, processes lights and sounds, sets the tone of your fight-or-flight response, and modulates your sensitivity to pain.

The middle and bottom parts of your brainstem– the pons and medulla, respectively, controls your heart rate and blood pressure, breathing, digestion and pain sensations in your head, face and jaw.

Clues that something's wrong:

Problems in your brainstem can lead to:

Scoring:

Place a 0, 1, 2 or 3 next to each symptom to grade its severity.

0 = none, 1 = mild, 2 = moderate and 3 = severe

Light and sound sensitivity	
Sleep disturbances	
Exaggeration startle response	
Sensitivity to pain	
Dizziness or migraine headaches	
Cold hands and feet	
Worsening of symptoms when reading a book or looking at a computer for very long	
Digestive symptoms - gas, bloating, SIBO, leaky gut	
High/low blood pressure	
Anxiety	
TOTAL SCORE	

NEURAL NETWORK #5: Inner Ear-Vestibular System

Where it's at:

Your inner ear is connected to a larger neural network called your vestibular system– that extends from inside your ear to deep within your brain.

What it does:

Its main job is to tell your brain where your head is relative to the rest of your body and the world around you, and to give you a real sense of grounding and balance.

Clues that something's wrong:

Damage to the inner ear and vestibular system is extremely common after a concussion and can lead to the following symptoms:

Scoring:

Place a 0, 1, 2 or 3 next to each symptom to grade its severity.

0 = none, 1 = mild, 2 = moderate and 3 = severe

Dizziness	
Vertigo	
Light headedness	
Balance problems	
Motion sickness	
Trouble walking up and down stairs	
Feeling anxious for no apparent reason	
Brief episodes of blurred vision	
A worsening of your symptoms when driving or with quick movements of your head	
A vague, floating feeling that something is just off, but very difficult to describe	
TOTAL SCORE	

So there you have it. The TOP 5 BrainSAVE! Neural Networks of Post-Concussion Syndrome. Like I mentioned before, there are many more neural networks and brain regions that can become damaged after a concussion, but these are the ones that I see most commonly in my practice and that can explain many of your post-concussion symptoms.

How to Identify Your Unique BrainSAVE! Imbalances

Now that you have a better understanding of the ROOT CAUSE for your symptoms, complete the following self-assessment QUIZ to identify your unique BrainSAVE! imbalances and to learn what you can do about them.

Self-Assessment QUIZ

Take the **Total Score** from each of the 5 BrainSAVE! Neural Networks and using the breakdown below, identify YOUR BrainSAVE! imbalances to find out what your next best actions are.

Score	Severity	Care Plan	Actions to Take
0-5	You may have a **MILD** imbalance in your Neural Networks	BrainSAVE! Self-Care	Complete the 6-Week Plan in Part III
6-10	You may have a **MODERATE** imbal-ance in your Neural Networks	BrainSAVE! Self-Care + **BrainSAVE! Exercises**	Complete the 6-Week Plan in Part III **Focus on the Brain-SAVE! Exercises in Week 3 of the 6-Week BrainSAVE! Plan**
11 and above	You may have a **SEVERE** imbalance in your Neural Networks	BrainSAVE! Self-Care + BrainSAVE! Exercises + **Medical Care**	Complete the 6-Week Plan in Part III Focus on the Brain-SAVE! Exercises in Week 3 of the 6-Week BrainSAVE! Plan **Apply for the 5-Day BrainSAVE! Recovery Program for Concussion**

What Happens to Your NEURAL NETWORKS after a Concussion?

Now that you've learned what neural networks are, the TOP 5 Brain-SAVE! Neural Networks, and which potential BrainSAVE! imbalances are at the ROOT CAUSE for your symptoms– let's take a deeper dive into what actually happens to your brain after a concussion. Because the following process is what causes your neural networks to weaken and break in the first place.

Immuno-toxici-WHAT??

In addition to the physical trauma of a head injury, there's also a chemical trauma that takes place. In many cases, this is what perpetuates and worsens the initial damage and leads to Post-Concussion Syndrome and CTE.

After a concussion, an **immune response** becomes triggered and immune cells known as microglia release powerful chemicals leading to widespread inflammation in your brain. If the levels of inflammation are high enough, brain cells can die.

When they die, they release other chemicals into the surrounding environment.

One of these is a chemical messenger called glutamate.

Glutamate is a very powerful excitatory neurotransmitter. When it makes contact with your brain cells, it tickles and stimulates them so they become activated. Normally, this happens in a very intentional and carefully regulated process.

If a brain cell dies from inflammation though, it randomly and haphazardly releases tons of glutamate into its surrounding environment. If nearby brain cells gobble up that glutamate, they too can become overstimulated and die.

This process is known as ***excitotoxicity***. Your brain cells are being literally tickled to death.

As you can see, a deadly chain reaction of inflammation and toxicity is triggered after a concussion– what neurologists call ***immunoexcitotoxicity***.[11]

If this process isn't put to a halt, it can lead to many of the symptoms of Post-Concussion Syndrome that you've been suffering from. And in some severe cases can lead to chronic traumatic encephalopathy.

There is serious damage being done to your neural networks and your brain begins to break.

INTERESTING TIDBIT

Mental and emotional traumas can trigger the same damaging chemical reaction in your brain as a physical trauma to your head!

BACK TO KAREN...

If there's too much inflammation in your frontal lobe guess what you'll experience? Brain fog, distractibility, mental fogginess, disorganized thought, forgetfulness and more.

This is what happened to Karen and was the ROOT CAUSE for her brain fog, forgetfulness, mental disorganization, ADD and the slowing of her eye movements.

If excitotoxicity happens in your cerebellum– you'll experience balance problems, clumsiness, chronic neck and back pain, and/or shaky hands

This was the ROOT CAUSE for Karen's dizziness and balance issues.

And if there's immunoexcitotoxicity happening in your vestibular system you may experience anxiety, dizziness, vertigo, light headedness, motion sickness, or feel out of sorts in a vague way that can be very hard to describe.

This was the ROOT CAUSE for Karen's anxiety, dizziness and motion sickness.

So now that you have a deeper understanding of the ROOT CAUSE for Post-Concussion Syndrome, have identified your own unique BrainSAVE! imbalances, and understand what happens to your brain after a concussion— the question that's probably on your mind is— *"So now what?"*.

CHAPTER 8

Introducing BrainSAVE!

FTER MANY YEARS OF RESEARCH, teaching doctors, seeing patients just like Karen, and healing my own concussed brain, I was able to put together a totally comprehensive, cutting-edge treatment program to address the ROOT CAUSE for Post-Concussion Syndrome, without the use of drugs or surgery.

Thus, was born the BrainSAVE! Recovery Program for Concussion.

The program is a 5-Day in-office intensive brain healing program based on the breakthrough scientific discoveries of neuroplasticity and epigenetics. The goal of the BrainSAVE! Recovery Program for Concussion is to REBUILD the broken neural networks that are the ROOT CAUSE for Post-Concussion Syndrome.

I've taken the most modern, state-of-the-art concussion therapies available today, combined them with ancient Eastern healing practices– and put them all together in a highly-personalized brain healing program.

It's an immersive brain training program that can dramatically accelerate the healing process. Many clients who go through the program report greater symptomatic relief after just 5 days– then they had experienced after all the months/years after their initial concussion.

When Karen was in town for her BrainSAVE! Program, I had her get some blood tests done to see if there were any other obstacles slowing down her recovery.

In the past when she would get her blood tested, she would literally pass out from her anxiety. This time was different though.

This time when she got her blood drawn, she barely even flinched! By precisely identifying the ROOT CAUSE for her Post-Concussion Syndrome we were able to dramatically lower her anxiety, clear her brain fog, decrease her dizziness and headaches by 70%, and eliminate her light and sound sensitivity by 85%– all within a matter of a few days of intensive treatments.

Seem like a miracle? I used to think so, especially when I first started seeing dramatic results like this years ago. But time after time, when patient after patient responded similarly, I knew I was on to something.

Since spaces for the 5-Day BrainSAVE! Program are limited, not everyone that applies gets accepted into the program– that's why I wrote this book for you and the millions of other people suffering from Post-Concussion Syndrome that may not be making it out to my center anytime soon. I want you to have access to this life-changing and cutting-edge information NOW, so you can begin your journey to great health TODAY.

I took the top actions, recommendations and brain rebuilding ex-ercises from my professional and personal experiences with concus-sion– and combined them all in the foundational 6-Week BrainSAVE! Plan that you will find in Part III of this book.

The 6-Week BrainSAVE! Plan is a collection of some of the most powerful actions that you can immediately take to begin healing your brain from your concussion, head injury, and brain trauma. The sug-gestions and recommendations will best prepare and PRIME your brain and body for the healing process.

And if you've already applied for and gotten accepted into the 5-Day BrainSAVE! Program, the 6-Week Plan is a great way to PRIME your brain cells for the state-of-the-art in-office BrainSAVE! concussion treatments that you'll be getting as part of your personalized 5-Day BrainSAVE! Program. Doing as much as you can of the 6-Week Plan will help you get the most out of your visit.

Before I walk you through all of the exciting details of the 6-Week Plan, I first need to bust apart a few myths about the brain and introduce you to the ground-breaking scientific discoveries that form the backbone of the BrainSAVE! method for treating Post-Concussion Syndrome without drugs or surgery.

PART II

Turning Myths into Miracles

CHAPTER 9

Myth Busting

Your Brain is Fixed

What you think, you become

—Buddha

T HE MAJORITY OF THE PATIENTS that come to my center after receiving a neurological diagnosis are worried, anxious, afraid and sometimes downright terrified.

And rightfully so.

Most of them don't think there's anything they can do to improve their situations, because they were taught that their brains are fixed, immutable and 100% under the control of genetics.

And that brain damage is irreversible.

In fact, many doctors still hold these false assumptions, even though the science and evidence tells a completely different story.[12]

Contrary to popular belief, your brain is not fixed. It is dynamic and mutable. And if there's damage to your neural networks, the damage can be reversed.

Your brain can and does heal.

Your brain has the remarkable ability to regenerate itself. You can strengthen existing connections in what is known as synaptic plasticity. You can forge new connections in a process called synaptogenesis. In fact, you can even grow new brain cells because of the miracle of neurogenesis.

So why aren't more doctors aware of this? Well, most of them are, in fact.

The concept of neuroplasticity– the amazing ability of your brain to change throughout your lifetime– is nothing new. Evidence for this phenomenon was discovered over 200 hundred years ago, by the Italian anatomist Michele Vicenzo Malacarne.

Still, as is the case with most revolutionary concepts, the majority of neuroscientists didn't widely accept this idea at first. The reigning paradigm of the day, until just recently, was that after a small window in early childhood, the brain was for the most part fixed and remained so for the rest of our lives.

But talk to anyone with any knowledge of the brain and they will all agree– the brain does change, based on our different experiences. Neuroplasticity is very real.

And this scientific breakthrough forms the foundation of my life's work– helping patients recover from chronic neurological conditions such as Post-Concussion Syndrome. And helping healthy people reach their highest spiritual, neurological and genetic potential. And it was through the miracle of neuroplasticity that I was able to heal my own brain.

The problem like I mentioned to you before is that there is usually a lag of about 20 years between scientific discoveries and real changes to the standard of care, and types of treatments being offered. Unfortunately, in the case of neuroplasticity, that lag has proven to be over 100 years!

And although most doctors *know about* neuroplasticity, there just aren't enough out there that know *what to do about it*[13], and *how to apply it to the care of their patients*[14]. Which is one of the main reasons why there are so many people still suffering from chronic neurological disorders such as Post-Concussion Syndrome.

But fear not. I'm bringing this information to you today, so that you can know WHAT you can do to start healing your brain now. I suffered from and healed my own broken brain– and in doing so discovered the secrets to healing and neuroplasticity in a very real way.

Why should any of this matter to you?

Because the way we will be addressing the ROOT CAUSE for your post-concussion symptoms is by taking advantage of this powerful concept of neuroplasticity[15]. Applying neuroplasticity to your life is how you'll be rebuilding your broken neural networks[16].

Let's take a closer look at what neuroplasticity is to help you better understand what I mean.

CHAPTER 10

The Miracle of Neuroplasticity

Experience coupled with attention leads to physical changes in the structure and future functioning of the nervous system. This leaves us with a clear, physiological fact...

Moment by moment we choose and sculpt how our ever-changing minds will work, we choose who we will be the next moment in a very real sense, and these choices are left embossed in physical form on our material selves.

–Dr. Michael Merzenich

Professor Emeritus, University of California

NEUROPLASTICITY IS YOUR BRAIN'S amazing ability to physically change its shape, size and structure– based on your different experiences. And when the structure of your brain changes, the function of your brain changes.

And when the function of your brain changes your experience of the world and of yourself changes.

This is what is known as *Experience-Dependent Neuroplasticity.*

Experience-Dependent Neuroplasticity[17] is how you were able to learn and get good at everything that you've done in your life – from walking, to riding your bike, to playing a musical instrument, to learning how to read, write, speak and understand language. All those things you learned growing up that are now second nature to you (or maybe not so second nature anymore, after your concussion!) happened because of Experience-Dependent Neuroplasticity.

When you were a toddler and just learning how to walk – all the sensory signals coming in from your muscles and joints and ligaments powerfully lit up and connected key neural networks related to balance, coordination and movement. And after doing it every single day for months and years, it started to become automatic. That wasn't muscle memory. That was the Cerebellar-Brainstem-Thalamic-Prefrontal Lobe Neural Network of Movement you were training.

That's Experience-Dependent Neuroplasticity.

And if you played the violin or some musical instrument like I did growing up, the gorgeous tones of the violin combined with the fine movements of my hands, fingers, and arms all sent small yet powerful electrical nerve signals that went zipping in through my ear and ear drum, past my brainstem, into my thalamus finally landing in the Temporal Lobe of my brain— where it was processed and experienced as that oh so glorious gift to us from the gods known as… music.

And the more I played and listened and practiced, the deeper and more refined my neural networks became[18]. I wasn't training my ears – I was training the Musical Neural Networks in my brain.

That's Experience-Dependent Neuroplasticity.

There are neural networks for focus, for reading, for pain relief, for being patient with your kids, for concentrating on your work, for creativity, for playing sports. And there are *Experience-Dependent Neuroplastic BrainSAVE! Treatments* that can specifically target and rebuild any neural networks that were damaged by a concussion. There are unique BrainSAVE! Treatments for each different neural network. For best results, you have to match the appropriate treatment to its respective network.

This is the scientific basis for the life-changing brain rebuilding treatments that I give to my patients to heal their brains[19], and what I did to heal my own brain.

And this is what I did with Karen to heal her brain.

Karen's Saga Continues...

If you recall, Karen's unique BrainSAVE! imbalances were:

1. Inner ear-Vestibular system
2. Prefrontal Cortex
3. Cerebellum

So a big part of Karen's treatment was geared towards retraining her inner ear and vestibular system through her senses.

My team and I used specific BrainSAVE! eye movement therapies[20], balance training, non-invasive cranial nerve stimulation, propriocep-tive retraining, vibration therapy, brain-boosting essential oils, concen-trated oxygen, and light therapy[21] – all with the goal of specifically tar-geting and rebuilding the weakened neural networks that were the ROOT CAUSE for her symptoms.

By identifying which of Karen's BrainSAVE! Neural Networks were broken and then matching it with the specific BrainSAVE! Treat-ments, I was able to put together her very own BrainSAVE! Protocol and dramatically reduce her anxiety, brain fog, dizziness, headaches, motion sickness, light and sound sensitivity and other post-concussion symptoms within a matter of days.

All of this was based on the revolutionary scientific discovery of Experience-Dependent Neuroplasticity.

Not all patients who do the 5-Day BrainSAVE! Program respond as quickly or as dramatically as Karen did. Everyone is neurologically unique and has different needs depending on their overall picture of health.

But I almost *always* see some level of improvement. Whether it's better balance and coordination, faster reaction time, pain relief, a deeper sense of calm. I welcome all of it as a cause for celebration. Because these are all signs of hope that the brain is healing. And with repeated treatments and at-home BrainSAVE! Exercises (some of which you'll be learning in Week 3 of the 6-Week BrainSAVE! Plan) the changes start to stick. And recovery becomes more long-term and permanent.

CHAPTER 11

It's All Connected

Knee bone connected to the –thigh bone–
Thigh bone connected to the –hip bone–
Hip bone connected to the –back bone–
Back bone connected to the –neck bone–
Neck bone connected to the –head bone–

–Dem Bones

James Weldon Johnson

THE PHENOMENON OF EXPERIENCE-DEPENDENT Neuroplasticity truly is a miracle and a gift to all of us who have brains. Which is everyone. You can use it to literally rebuild the connections between your broken neural networks, fix your brain, and live the life of your imagination and design.

But on the other hand– if you eat a crappy diet, have loads of unmanaged stress, and are running on empty all the time– no matter how much work you put into rebuilding your neural networks, you'll be taking one step forward and three steps back.

Because it's all connected.

One of the main reasons why Karen responded so well to her treatments was because she had done a lot of the necessary groundwork at home to PRIME her brain, before flying in for her 5-Day BrainSAVE! Program. She took action on and followed through with many of the same juicy tips and recommendations that you'll be learning in the 6-Week BrainSAVE! Plan that's included in this book.

And Karen's response to care is pretty typical. In my practice, I witness anything from slow and steady improvements over time, to immediate and instantaneous transformations– and everything in between.

But in the past, when I was figuring all this out– I had a small yet significant number of patients who even after months of weekly in-office brain rebuilding treatments failed to get very far with their care.

And just like I do with all my patients, I did what I was born to do. I dove deeper and asked WHY. Why weren't they responding to care like everyone else? Why weren't they getting better? Why weren't their brains healing?

And I would explore their histories with them in greater depth, asking them better questions, trying to understand the unique situations surrounding their health. And over time I began to see some very specific patterns.

These patterns also explained why some people develop post-concussion syndrome and CTE after a head injury and some don't. And why the severity of the concussion doesn't always match up with the severity of the concussion symptoms.

You probably know some people who had experienced some pretty bad head injuries and yet they seem totally fine now. And maybe your concussion didn't even feel that bad at the time but yet here you are, struggling after all these months and years.

Why?

More likely than not, one or more of the following 12 Obstacles to Healing was present at or around the time of your concussion– preventing your brain from fully recovering.

So without further ado– read on to discover the 12 Biggest Obstacles to Healing from Post-Concussion Syndrome that I've identified over the years.

CHAPTER 12

The 12 Biggest Obstacles to Healing

THE 12 BIGGEST OBSTACLES TO Healing from Post-Concussion Syndrome:

1. Unchecked brain inflammation

2. Unmanaged mental and emotional stress

3. Digestive imbalances

4. Blood sugar imbalances

5. Sensitive mitochondria

6. Food sensitivities

7. Hormone imbalances

8. Joint and muscular imbalances

9. Toxins

10. Single nucleotide polymorphisms

11. Untreated autoimmune diseases

12. Hidden infections

An in-depth discussion of each these 12 obstacles is way beyond the scope of this book, but I wanted to list them here for you so you can become aware of them. Because the good news is, that once the obstacle is identified and removed, your broken neural networks can come back to life again.

Your brain can finally heal.

Self-Assessment QUIZ

Find out if one or more of the 12 Obstacles to Healing are impacting your concussion recovery by taking the following QUIZ. Check the boxes if you can relate to any of the following:

Obstacles to Healing QUIZ

You have a degenerative health condition like thyroid disease, diabetes, autoimmune, chronic fatigue syndrome in addition to PCS	☐
You have degenerative diseases on your mom's side of the family	☐
You get lightheaded and/or hangry if you haven't eaten recently	☐
You get sleepy or tired after you eat	☐
You have gas, bloating, diarrhea, constipation, leaky gut or SIBO	☐
You have a hard time falling asleep and/or staying asleep	☐
You've taken more than one course of antibiotics throughout your life	☐
You don't have any consistent stress management practices or time for relaxation	☐
You easily tire and get fatigued after exercising	☐
You experience pain and tightness in your muscles and joints	☐
You have unexplained itchy skin, rashes or bumps	☐
You have symptoms around your period if you're a woman or early balding or erectile dysfunction if you're a man	☐

Scoring the QUIZ

Score one point for each box you checked.

Score	Severity	Actions to Take
0-4	There is a **slight** possibility that one or more of these obstacles is keeping your brain from healing.	Complete the 6-Week Plan in Part III
5+	There is a **high** likelihood that one or more of these obstacles is keeping your brain from healing.	1) Complete the 6-Week Plan in Part III 2) Apply for a Comprehensive Modern BrainEVAL so you can learn which of these obstacles is keeping your brain from healing and WHAT you can do to about it.

You can also try to find a Functional Medicine doctor that specializes in neurology and work with them to help you identify which of these obstacles is keeping you from healing (see Brain-Boosting Resources).

Either way, the good news is that since it's all connected, when you remove one obstacle, many of the other ones will begin to shift as well. So by following the recommendations in the 6-Week BrainSAVE! Plan 100%, you will already be addressing several of the major obstacles.

But if you've done the plan 100% as recommended and still aren't feeling much better, then I highly encourage you to seek out the services of a trained professional who understands the big picture of neurology and Functional Medicine and work with them to unravel your case.

And if you're having neck and spinal issues, find yourself a good, gentle chiropractor or osteopath to make sure your spine is in great alignment and that the core of your nervous system is solid.

Or if you're not sure what foods are good and bad for your brain, look for a nutritionist or health coach who can help you eat right for your brain type (see Brain-Boosting Resources).

And finally, it may be a good idea to seek out the services of a massage therapist that can help ease the tension in your muscles and joints.

It's just that important. *You're that important.*

Because even the presence of just one of these obstacles can be enough to keep your brain from ever fully recovering from your concussion.

PART III

The 6-Week BrainSAVE! Plan

Overview of the 6-Week Plan

Now that you've learned about the ROOT CAUSE for your post-concussion symptoms, identified your broken BrainSAVE! Neural Networks, learned about Experience-Dependent Neuroplasticity, and discovered the biggest obstacles to healing, you're probably asking yourself, *"So what can I do about it?"*

That's where the 6-Week BrainSAVE! Plan comes in.

I've taken some of the most powerful actions and lessons from the 5-Day BrainSAVE! Program and laid it out for you in a 6-Week Plan to heal your brain from concussions, brain injuries and trauma.

Goal of the Plan

The 6-Week BrainSAVE! Plan is intended to activate your brain's natural ability to heal itself. It's meant to PRIME your brain for healing– by decreasing neuroinflammation, supporting your mitochondria, calming immunoexcitotoxicity, enhancing detoxification, expanding your mind, and sparking your neuroepigenetic potential for rebuilding your neural networks.

6-Week Overview

Week 1: PRIME YOUR CELLS

Week 2: PUT OUT THE FIRE

Week 3: REBUILD

Week 4: SLOW DOWN

Week 5: TAKE OUT THE TRASH

Week 6: EXPAND YOUR MIND

Imagine each week as a stepping stone out of the mire of pain and suffering and into the light of healing and recovery. Here's some of what you'll be learning:

- The BrainSAVE! Food Plan
- Top 5 BrainSAVE! Supplements
- 7 Foundational BrainSAVE! Exercises
- Key BrainSAVE! Lifestyle Strategies
- BrainSAVE! Visualization Exercise
- And more!

Now that you have a better idea of what the plan looks like, let's dive right in!

The 6-Week BrainSAVE! Plan
to Heal Your Brain
from Concussions,
Brain Injuries & Trauma

WEEK 1: PRIME YOUR CELLS

Welcome to the first day of the rest of your life!

The purpose of Week 1 of your 6-Week BrainSAVE! Plan is to begin priming your brain cells for the brain rebuilding exercises you'll be starting in Week 3. The main actions you'll be taking this week are:

1. Starting your BrainSAVE! Supplements
2. Starting your BrainSAVE! Keto Shake
3. Reading labels and asking questions
4. Getting rid of gluten

BrainSAVE! Supplements

Supplements are a really important part of the BrainSAVE! approach to Post-Concussion Syndrome. They are a safe and fast way to increase levels of nutrients that the brain needs to heal after a concussion.

I usually put my patients on a variety of different supplements at the start of care, depending on their level of inflammation, overall health and pre-existing conditions– as well as the results of their advanced Functional Medicine testing.

Talk to your doctor to find the right dosage for you based on your weight, age, and or other personal health issues.

That being said here are the TOP 5 BrainSAVE! Supplements for you to start taking now.

1. High quality DHA supplement

DHA is a fatty acid that's found in high concentrations in your brain membranes. It allows for neuronal communication, decreases inflammation and turns on the gene that produces BDNF– a protein that is essential for neuroplasticity.

2. Magnesium threonate

Magnesium is a master mineral that's involved in over 300 enzymatic reactions in your brain and body, yet it is one of the most common mineral deficiencies in the United States. Magnesium supports neuroplasticity and is able to stabilize unstable brain cells that are feeling a bit immunoexcitotoxic after a concussion.

When attached to a molecule known as threonate, the two have been shown to easily cross the blood brain barrier, making it more available to calm your frazzled brain cells.

3. Liposomal glutathione

Glutathione is your brain's master antioxidant. It powerfully quenches free radicals and protects your brain cells and mitochondria from damaging toxins. Liposomes protect it from being broken down by your digestive system, so more can reach the cells and mitochondria in your brain.

4. Ginkgo biloba

Ginkgo biloba has been used in Chinese medicine for over 5000 years. It improves circulation to brain cells, protects the brain from stress-induced cell death and turns on the gene that makes glutathione.

5. Curcumin

Curcumin is a polyphenol found in the spice turmeric, that gives it that rich, bold, yellow color. It has been used in Chinese and Indian medicine for thousands of years and is a very powerful natural anti-inflammatory compound.

NOT ALL SUPPLEMENTS ARE CREATED EQUAL

There isn't much regulation of supplements by the FDA. I have mixed feelings about that. On the one hand, you don't need a prescription from a doctor to get vitamins. But on the other hand, you can't be sure of the safety and quality of the supplements that you are getting.

Over the course of many years, I've curated the highest quality supplements from several companies that I completely trust-ones that I personally take every day, recommend to my family and friends, and prescribe to all my patients with great results (visit bit.ly/brainsavesupps). So be sure to do your research before buying random supplements online or at a health food store.

BrainSAVE! Keto Shake

Breakfast is the most important meal of the day. It sets the tone of your metabolism for the rest of your day. Most people (myself included before I learned about how to better care for my brain) go about their day without eating anything in the morning.

Or if they do have breakfast it consists of a lot of sugar and un-healthy carbs– cereal with milk, bagel with orange juice, toast with jam. Yummy, but very high in refined sugars that can thwart the healing process and cause massive inflammation in your brain and body.

This BrainSAVE! Keto Shake is great because it's simple to make, tastes great, is low in sugar, and high in healthy fats– which your brain thrives on. Play around with the ratios if it's too creamy, or too bitter, or too sour for your tastes until you get it just right.

Here's the recipe:

BRAINSAVE! KETO SHAKE

Organic ingredients:

1-2 avocados
1 stalk of celery
1/2 cucumber
1 peeled lemon
1/2 bunch of parsley
8-12 leaves of fresh basil
½ cup of virgin coconut oil
1/3 cup of extra virgin olive oil
2 cups of pure water
Dash of pink Himalayan sea salt

Directions:

Blend all the brain-healing ingredients together in a Vitamix or blender.

Add ice/water and salt to taste.

Makes 2-3 servings

Reading Labels and Asking Questions

If you're not already, start reading labels at the grocery store and start asking questions when eating out about the following foods:

1. Gluten
2. Dairy
3. Sugar
4. Excitotoxins
    a. MSG
    b. Hydrolyzed vegetable protein
    c. Yeast extract
    d. Aspartame
    e. Artificial sweeteners and colors
5. Other chemicals

If you can't pronounce it with your tongue, don't put it on your tongue– or eat it with your mouth!

Become aware of and familiar with which foods contain gluten, dairy, added sugars, excitotoxins and other brain-draining chemicals.

Getting Rid of Gluten

If there is one dietary tweak that you're going to make that will have the most powerful impact on your recovery, it's this– STOP EATING GLUTEN.

Gluten, a protein found in yummy foods such as cakes, cookies, bread, pasta, and pizza, has been scientifically shown to destroy the brains[22], cerebellums[23], and nerves[24] of people who are sensitive to it. And I'll have to tell you– 99% of ALL the patients that I've worked with over the years had a sensitivity to gluten one degree or another. And it wasn't until they removed it completely that their brains began to heal.

I found this to be true for myself as well. For years, I knew about gluten sensitivity. I studied it, I researched it, I prescribed gluten-free diets to my patients. I even experimented with going gluten-free myself. And I definitely felt better so I stayed at about 80% gluten-free for many years. But after learning more and more about the horrible effects that gluten had on the brain, I decided to go 100% gluten-free.

That decision saved my life. Many of the darker, psychological symptoms that I had been suffering from such as anger, depression, worry, irritability, brain fog completely lifted. I was sold.

So if there's only one change to your diet that you'll be making during the next six weeks, I strongly suggest you get rid of gluten.

WEEK 2: PUT OUT THE FIRE

Now that you've PRIMED your brain cells with key brain-boosting nutrients and supplements, as well as gotten rid of GLUTEN– one of the biggest causes of unchecked inflammation, it's time to really put out the fire in your brain.

Here are the main actions you'll be taking this week:

1. Continue your BrainSAVE! Supplements
2. Get rid of ALL inflammatory foods from your diet
    a. Gluten
    b. Dairy
    c. Refined sugars
    d. Excitotoxins
    e. Processed foods
3. Eat more brain supporting foods

Foods to Eat and Avoid

AVOID

1. Remove ALL excitotoxins from your diet
   a. Most fast food and processed food uses some form of MSG, not just Chinese food so continue to ask questions and read labels.
2. Remove all gluten, dairy and refined sugar from your diet.
3. Avoid soda, fruit juice, energy drinks and choose spring water, sparkling water, tea and low-sugar veggie drinks instead.

Almost every time I've given this sad news to my patients, the usual response is, *"Then what can I eat???"*, spoken with big bulging eyeballs in a tone of despair, overwhelm and fear.

Fear not!

The BrainSAVE! Food Plan is a healthy mix of Paleo-Ketogenic-Mediterranean. It's full of lean meats, healthy fats, minimal fruit, a few nuts and seeds– with a LOT of low carb veggies. Think nutrient-dense, organic, pesticide-free, healthy, delicious.

There are a LOT of yummy foods that you can eat on this plan.

Here's a few of them:

EAT

Loads of healthy fats. Your brain is 60% fat. So fatten it up:

- Coconut oil
- Olives
- Olive oil
- Avocados
- Guacamole
- Nuts and seeds

A lot of low carb veggies – at least 4-6 servings a day:

- Cabbage
- Broccoli
- Asparagus
- Romanesco broccoli
- Romaine lettuce
- Cucumbers
- Celery
- Artichoke
- Chives
- Watercress
- Pea shoots
- Sprouts

Moderate amounts of protein – about the size of your palm for each meal:

- SMASH fish
    - Sardines, mackerel, anchovies, salmon and herring
- Meat
    - Beef, buffalo, elk, lamb, venison
    - Chicken, duck, turkeys
    - Grass-fed, organic sources are best
- Beans, small amounts of tofu, chickpeas

Some low-glycemic, brain-nourishing fruits – 1-2 servings a day:

- Blueberries
- Kiwis
- Cherries
- Berries
- Apple
- Pomegranate seeds

Healthy nuts and seeds – no more than a handful a day:

- Cashews
- Almonds
- Walnuts
- Macadamia nuts
- Brazil nuts
- Flax seeds
- Pumpkin seeds
- Chia seeds
- Sesame seeds

What to Expect...

At the end of week 2, you might start feeling better already. If you've followed along and have implemented everything from weeks 1 and 2, here are some things you may be experiencing: less fogginess, more energy, better sleep, better bowel movements. Not bad for only two weeks on the plan huh?

But you might actually be feeling worse, due to withdrawal or blood-sugar dips and shifts. That's a common response as well.

Stick with it. If you get hungry or hangry, be sure you're getting enough healthy fats in your diet and/or eating enough low carb veggies. Snack on these when you feel lightheaded or hungry or are craving sugary foods or junk food.

Getting tired of the same old same old?

Here is a great recipe and meal planning app we absolutely love and recommend to all of our patients who need a little more help coming up with creative and delicious brain-nourishing meal ideas (visit Real Plans at www.realplans.com, also noted in Brain-Boosting Resources).

Bon appétit!

WEEK 3: REBUILD

Now that you've done a lot of the groundwork in Weeks 1 and 2, this is where the fun part begins. The purpose of Week 3 is to REBUILD YOUR NEURAL NETWORKS with Experience-Dependent Neuro-plasticity– the whole reason for PRIMING your brain cells in the first place.

The main actions you'll be taking are the 7 Foundational Brain-SAVE! Exercises to REBUILD your neural networks:

1. BrainSAVE! Balance exercise
2. BrainSAVE! Tooth Brushing
3. Vagal Rinse
4. Splash 'n Calm
5. Figure-8

6. Frontal Lobe Finger Tap

7. Temporal Tonic

Personal training for your brain

If you had a goal of getting healthy and losing weight and building muscles, you might see a nutritionist who would customize a meal plan for you, maybe recommend some vitamins and supplements. If the program was right for your unique genetic make-up, you would most likely lose weight.

But what about building muscles or toning up? That wouldn't happen unless you actually did some physical exercise as well– push-ups, pull ups, lifting weights. That's what Week 3 is all about– toning and sculpting your brain by using your body, your senses and Experience-Dependent Neuroplasticity.

This is where you'll start REBUILDING your weakened neural networks. Like I mentioned in chapter 10, you can activate and strengthen your neural networks by using your senses, just like you did when you were a little baby exploring the world.

The good news is that you've already built them before, when you were growing up from infant, to toddler, to little kid, to young adult to where you were at before your head injury– so it should be easier this time around.

And it shouldn't take as long either to regain your balance, your focus, your confidence, your energy and your reaction time. Although your neural networks may be a bit scrambled after your concussion, the miracle of neuroplasticity will allow you to rewire your brain and rewrite your life.

At my integrative neurology center, I use countless BrainSAVE! treatments and state-of-the-art brain-healing technologies to accelerate my patients' recovery, each one personalized to their unique neural network imbalance:

- Specific eye exercises[25]– the direction, speed, and size of the movements can specifically target different neural networks that are unique to your neurological needs
- Laser guided eye movements – using the latest technologies I can further refine the precision of the treatment
- Low level laser therapy[26] – to decrease neuroinflammation and boost mitochondrial function
- Infrared Sauna Therapy[27] – to improve brain circulation and safely enhance detoxification
- Transcutaneous Cranial Nerve Stimulation[28] – to non-invasively stimulate brainstem neural networks
- Brain-Boosting Essential Oil Therapy – to target key neural networks related to memory, mood and cognition
- Rebound therapy – to improve lymphatic drainage and to activate your inner ear-vestibular neural network

- BrainSAVE! Vestibular Rehab[29] – to rebuild the neural networks related to balance, dizziness and vertigo
- And more

That being said here are the 7 Foundational BrainSAVE! Exercises you can do on your own at home, to begin rebuilding your brain. I designed these so they can be easily incorporated into your everyday life.

1. **BrainSAVE! Balance exercise**
   - To do this exercise, first you'll need to find out which foot is wobblier
   - Balance on your left foot for as long as you can
   - Now, balance on your right foot for as long as you can
   - Which foot was wobblier? If both were pretty solid, try doing it with your eyes closed.
   - If your left foot was wobblier, your job is to balance on your left foot. If your right foot was wobblier, your job is to balance on your right foot.
     - o Set a goal for 30 seconds without having to put your other foot down for balance. Once you hit that, go up to 60 seconds. You can make it more challenging by closing your eyes
     - o Do it once in the morning and once in the evening

o This BrainSAVE! exercise will REBUILD the brain cells in your Cerebellum and Inner Ear-Vestibular system

2. BrainSAVE! Tooth Brushing

- Movement is very much tied up with the strength and development of your Frontal and Prefrontal Lobes
- For the rest of the 6 weeks, simply brush your teeth with your non-dominant hand
  - o If you're right handed, use your left hand and vice versa
- Do this exercise twice a day
- This BrainSAVE! exercise will help strengthen your frontal lobe, on the opposite side of the hand you're using to brush your teeth with i.e. left hand = right frontal lobe

3. Vagal Rinse

- The muscles that control your throat and soft palate are controlled by neurons in your brainstem, so when you exercise your soft palate muscles, you exercise your brainstem. Here's what you'll do:
  - o After you've brushed your teeth, I want you to gargle using warm water
  - o Your goal is to be able to gargle for 60 seconds straight
  - o If you can't do it for the entire time, then spit out and continue where you left off

      o Do it once in the morning and once in the evening

- This will help activate your vagus nerve located in your brain-stem– a very important part of your parasympathetic nervous system – the one that allows you to rest, digest, feel calm and to heal.

- In all the patients that I've worked with over the years, every single one of them had a fight-or-flight response that was stuck in overdrive to varying degrees. Any little stressor– light, sound, emotion, feeling, movement would kick it further into overdrive. This will help reset that.

4. **Splash 'n Calm**

- After you've done your Vagal Rinse you'll be doing the Splash 'n Calm

- You do this by simply splashing cold water on your face. But really cold water. So cold that you're almost to the point of pain, but not quite.

- This also helps activate the vagus nerve and over time will reset your fight-or-flight response

- Repeat for a total of 5 times

5. **Figure-8**

- Coordinated, flowing movements are one of the most powerful ways to activate your Cerebellum and Prefrontal Cortex

- To do this rebuilding exercise, you're going to have to find out which is your most uncoordinated arm – the left or the right

- o Make figure-8 patterns with your left arm, focusing on movement at your shoulder
- o Repeat using your right arm
- o Whichever arm was the most uncoordinated is the one you'll be doing the Figure-8 with
- Trace figure-8 movements with your arm for one minute, three times a day
- If both are pretty uncoordinated, then do both, one at a time
- This exercise will help REBUILD and HEAL both your Cerebellum and your Frontal lobe

6. **Frontal Lobe Finger Tap**

- This is a very powerful meditation drawn from Kundalini yoga practices that has been shown to powerfully activate your Prefrontal Cortex[30].
- For this BrainSAVE! exercise you are going to be tapping your fingers together 4 times in this pattern:
  1) Thumb to index
  2) Thumb to middle finger
  3) Thumb to ring finger
  4) Thumb to pinky
- As you tap, you are going to be repeating the words "Saa, taa, naa, maa" for each finger you tap. For example, when you tap your thumb to your index, you'll say "Saa". When you tap your thumb to middle finger, you'll say "Taa", and so on and so forth.

- Once you've tapped all four finger and said "Saa, taa, naa, maa", you'll start the cycle over by tapping your thumb to your index again.
- Do it with both your left and your right hand. If you find one side is harder to do, then focus on only doing that side, until it becomes easier. You can then do both sides together again.
- Do this for 5 minutes, twice a day.
- You can also do this while you're walking for added benefit.

7. **Temporal Tonic**

   - If you have sensitivity to sound and/or a Temporal Lobe neural network imbalance, you will love this exercise. You'll need ear plugs and in-ear headphones– one to dampen sounds, and the other to increase sounds
   - To do this exercise, you're going to have to find out which ear is the most sensitive to sound. In many situations, you'll find that although both may be sensitive, there is usually one of them that is more so than the other. You can do this by playing music loudly on your phone and then bringing it up to your left ear, and then to your right. One side should feel more sensitive/irritating.
   - Here's what you'll do: wear the ear plug in the more sensitive ear for 30 minutes, three times a day. At the same time, listen to music using your in-ear headphones in the opposite ear. If that ear is also sensitive to sound, then do it at the lowest volume you can tolerate.

- If both ears are just as sensitive to sound, here's what you'll do: listen to music on the same side as your wobbly foot, and plug your opposite ear. For example, if your left foot was wobbly, listen to music in your left ear and plug your right.

- Doing this will calm your overactive brainstem and activate an underactive Temporal Lobe and balance your BrainSAVE! Neural Networks.

There you have it! The 7 Foundational BrainSAVE! Exercises to heal and REBUILD your broken neural networks. Here they are again for your viewing pleasure:

1. BrainSAVE! Balance exercise
2. BrainSAVE! Tooth Brushing
3. Vagal Rinse
4. Splash 'n Calm
5. Figure-8
6. Frontal Lobe Finger Tap
7. Temporal Tonic

Just like building muscles, the more you do these exercises over time, the stronger your neural networks will become.

Personalization is KEY

Personalization can really make all the difference in your recovery– you want to be sure you're matching the perfect BrainSAVE! Treatment with your unique BrainSAVE! Neural Network imbalance. So if you're not seeing much improvement after six weeks on the program, I encourage you to apply for a Comprehensive Modern BrainEVAL (see Brain-Boosting Resources). You can also try to find a Functional Neurologist in your area who specializes in Post-Concussion Syndrome, so they can help personalize a treatment plan that's right for your unique neural network imbalances.

Stack 'em!

When I'm working with patients at my integrative brain center, I like to stack several different BrainSAVE! treatments together at the same time. This powerfully activates the specific broken neural network combinations that are unique to their ROOT CAUSE– giving them faster and longer lasting results.

Once you get good at the different BrainSAVE! Exercises, have fun with it and start stacking them together. For example, once you're able to balance on your wobbly foot for 60 seconds straight, try doing that while doing the BrainSAVE! Tooth Brushing *and* Temporal Tonic at the same time.

Or once you've gotten more coordinated with Figure-8, try doing that PLUS the Frontal Lobe Finger Tap at the same time, *while* balancing on your wobbly foot.

Not only does this keep things fun, challenging and interesting for you, it's also a really important part of the healing process. Because when you stack the BrainSAVE! Exercises together, not only are you getting better at balancing on one leg and doing funky arm and finger movements. More importantly, you're creating Experience-Dependent Neuroplasticity and strengthening the connections between your Cerebellar–Prefrontal Cortex–Inner Ear-Vestibular System BrainSAVE! Neural Networks– all at the same time!

The combinations for stacking are endless.

Progress, NOT perfection

As with anything in life, it's not about perfection. It's about PROGRESS. We're looking for steady, gradual improvement over time.

Because when these BrainSAVE! Exercises become easier for you and you're able to do them for longer, and it becomes second nature– it doesn't just mean that your fingers are getting stronger, or your leg is getting steadier or your arms more coordinated– it's an objective sign and proof that your BrainSAVE! Neural Networks are healing! How cool is that?

WEEK 4: SLOW DOWN

In weeks 1-3 you started your supplements, changed up your diet and began your BrainSAVE! Exercises to rebuild your brain. Great job! That's a lot to take on. You may be feeling a bit overwhelmed at this point, with all the big changes and brain exercises that you've been doing the past 3 weeks.

And for that reason, I designed week 4 to give you and your brain a break.

The main actions you'll be taking this week are:

1. ………….
2. ………….
3. ………….

Nothing! That's right, this week is all about slowing down, resting and recuperating, and doing NOTHING. Here's how we're going to go about doing nothing:

1. Getting enough sleep
2. BrainSAVE! mini-breaks

Getting enough sleep

I know, I know– many of you reading this are probably thinking to yourself– I haven't had a good night's sleep in ages, after my head injury. There are many physiological reasons for that and ways of getting to the ROOT CAUSE, but it's still important to do the best you can and create the best environment and hygiene to get the best sleep you can. Because when you sleep at night, your brain's detoxification systems kick into high gear and flushes out your brain's excess gunk.[31] And the less deep, quality sleep you get, more and more toxic proteins begin to accumulate in your brain, mucking up your neural networks.

Here are some simple steps you can take to help improve your sleep:

*   Follow the 2-hour rule
    o   Dim or turn off the majority of the lights in your house 2 hours before bedtime

- o Use special filters on your smartphone or computer to block out harmful lights that mess up your circadian rhythm
  - ▪ F.lux is the one that I use for my computer.
  - ▪ Your smartphone should also have an automatic sleep/dimmer mode that you can preset
- o Turn ALL electronics off 1 hour before bedtime.
- o Instead, use a candle, read a book, listen to soft relaxing music, do gentle stretching, meditate, practice yoga, take a bath, make sweet love, journal to ease your mind or anything else that doesn't require a lot of mental activity and/or bright lights/electronics
- Create a sleep cave
  - o Get rid of any excess light in your bedroom. You may want to consider purchasing blackout curtains, or a sleep mask.
  - o Other sources of light are alarm clocks, night lights etc.

Downtime

In addition to sleep, one of the most important things you can do to heal your brain is having enough DOWNTIME. Especially for those of you who aren't able to get a good night's sleep because of pain, headaches or the fact that any little noise wakes up you at night.

I see this every single day. One of the biggest mistakes my concussion patients make when getting started, or when trying to navigate the confusing waters of TBI, is doing too much. And not taking enough time to rest and recuperate.

Or trying to push through even if their brains and bodies are telling them STOP! I totally get that. You want to do as much as you were able to do, think as fast as you were able to think before your head injury.

And so this next BrainSAVE! Lifestyle Strategy that you'll be learning is perhaps one of the most important ones for you to let marinate and simmer. And it's this– it's okay to slow down, stop and silently smell the roses. In fact, it's absolutely essential for the healing process, and to allow the magic of neuroplasticity to take hold.[32]

It doesn't mean you have to completely stop everything and not have a life.

But then again, depending on the severity of your concussion and how much your neural networks were altered or how much inflammation you have you might very well have to do that for a certain period of time.

But if you don't have that luxury, then this next (non) exercise can be a lifesaver for you.

Here's what you'll do:

BrainSAVE! mini-breaks

Start taking **BrainSAVE! mini-breaks** throughout the day. Every 30-60 minutes, I want you to begin taking little mini vacations from your life. This will allow your brain to reset and clear the junk that's built up between your synapses. Your mini-break can be anywhere from 1 minute to half an hour.

Heck if you really need to and have the luxury, go ahead and take a nap while you're at it. Just set your alarm as needed.

The important thing with mini-breaks is to check in with yourself. Are you talking to someone and just can't follow their train of thought, or your head starts hurting? Take a breather. Let them know you're reaching synaptic saturation.

Or you're reading this book, and you feel dizzy or nauseous. That's okay. Take a break.

Or you just can't handle driving with all the movement and light and you're feeling overwhelmed. Well guess what? It's okay to pull over.

We are so trained in our hectic modern world to keep going and going, doing and doing with no time left for being or healing. This week is all about being and healing.

Because without DOWNTIME and restorative practices, there is no way that your brain will be able to heal.

I know, I know– it sucks! What you used to be able to do in 5 minutes now takes an hour if you can even do it. And I know I know you don't want to rest. It's not fair. Yeah– you're right. Life ain't fair. But it is what it is so time to tough it out and…..

Stop.

Chill out.

Close your eyes.

Breathe.

Gently rub your eyeballs.

Or stretch, yawn, go for a little walk around the block, and find somewhere quiet to recharge if needed– let your body do what it already knows it needs to do.

The key is that these mini-breaks have to be unstructured, with no focus on tasks at hand whatsoever. That means no social media, no smartphone, Facebook, Instagram, TV, a mentally/emotionally heavy conversation, or anything that requires much mental energy at all.

You'll know you're doing it right when you find yourself feeling less fatigued throughout the day, or don't have to crash as hard at night or over the weekend. The paradoxical thing is that the more DOWNTIME you have doing NOTHING, the more charged and energized you become in your life.

This is one of the most important lessons you can take from this entire 6-Week BrainSAVE! Plan and bring with you into your life, even after you've healed from your head injury.

So really take the time to sit and do NOTHING.

WEEK 5: TAKE OUT THE TRASH

At this point in the program you've already done a good job decreasing inflammation by eating more foods that feed your brain and avoiding foods that cause damage. You've been taking your supplements. You've been rebuilding your neural networks with your BrainSAVE! exercises. And you've been giving yourself adequate DOWNTIME to allow the networks to thrive and grow, and for your brain to heal.

Now it's time to go in and get rid of any leftover trash. In your body, in your brain and in your mind.

The main actions you'll be taking are:

1. Eating cleansing foods
2. Sweating

3. Drinking pure water

4. Going on a BrainSAVE! Digital Detox

We live in a toxic world. The Environmental Working Group found an average of 200 industrial chemicals and pollutants in the umbilical cords of infants born in the US.[33]

And the types of toxins we're exposed to these days we never even came face to face with throughout our entire history on this planet.

So why aren't we all dead? The good news is that it's not just the amount of toxins we're exposed to that determines our health, it's the toxins in minus the toxins out.

The wonderful thing is that all throughout nature there are foods and plants and herbs that contain natural powerful chemicals that help rid our body of excess toxins. Many of the veggies I recommended in week 2 such as broccoli, asparagus, artichoke, chives, watercress and pea shoots have these already built in so eat more of these and eat from the rainbow.

Sweat, Drink, Digital Detox

Here are some more actions you can take this week to help you take out the trash.

1.   Sweat more. And often. If you're not able to exercise as much, try using a sauna, but don't go too long to avoid passing out. Start at 5 minutes and ease your way up.

    •   We have an infrared sauna at our integrative neurology practice that we regularly use and recommend for our patients because it has been shown to greatly enhance the removal of toxins, much more than just through regular sweat alone.

    •   Many patients of mine end up buying their own saunas since they love it so much. Here's the one that we use in our practice and highly recommend: : bit.ly/sunlightenKOBA

2.   Drink loads of pure water

    •   Start with ½ liter of filtered water with freshly squeezed lemon juice first thing in the morning

    •   Sip more throughout the day

    •   Your goal is to go to the bathroom every two hours, so that your urine is clear and odorless.

3.   Go on a BrainSAVE! Digital Detox

BrainSAVE! Digital Detox

I know I know but that's all you have now to keep yourself from going crazy but trust me, this will go a long way's towards saving your brain AND your sanity:

- Cut the amount of time you're on your smartphone or computer in half
- Take BrainSAVE! mini-breaks from your smartphone, computer or TV every 30-60 minutes when you do use them
- Schedule a time in your calendar to go on a one-week digital detox
    - No internet, no Facebook, Instagram, email unless you absolutely need it for work or crucial communication
    - Choose books, meditation, listening to or playing music, writing, painting, drawing, journaling, baths, stretching, yoga, walks around the block, and fun conversations with family and friends instead

WEEK 6: EXPAND YOUR MIND

Yes! You've made it this far! Only one more week to go.

So far, you've laid a great foundation for brain health and healing: you've primed your cells, put out the fire of brain inflammation, began rebuilding your neural networks, slowed down and taken out the trash.

Now you can begin to reap the rewards of all your hard work (and non-work you did in Week 4!). In this sixth and final week of the Brain-SAVE! Plan, you will be taking advantage of your minds uncanny ability to REBUILD your brain. In doing so, you will be rewriting the course of your brain injury, and your life.

You will tap into the power of your thoughts and imagination to visualize the health and healing that you want in your life with this

BrainSAVE! Visualization.

Here's what you'll do:

Find a calm and quiet place, separate from all the normal hustle and bustle of your daily life. I don't recommend your bedroom, but if that's the only place you can have some peace and quiet, that will suffice.

Gently close your eyes and meditate on this question: *What do I want my health for?*

Whatever comes to mind, allow it to be. If nothing happens, ask yourself that question again. Is it to spend more quality time with your kids? Or to be more patient with them? To graduate from school? To be able to start your own business? Or maybe so you can play music again, write your first book, or get back to playing sports? There is no right or wrong answer here, only what is true to your heart.

Now imagine yourself already in that place, already having achieved your health goals for this purpose.

What does it feel like? What do you see? Hear? Smell? What emotions are you experiencing? Steep in the experience of all of it as deeply as you can. Breathe deeply and let it all sink in.

At first, it may be difficult for you to sit in silence with your eyes closed trying to focus in silence, let alone visualize a future reality where you've already achieved your health goals. That's okay. Because by the nature of how Experience-Dependent Neuroplasticity works, the more you practice this, the easier and more effective it will become.

Feel free to use music or white noise, or to diffuse some essential oils like lavender or grapefruit that relax you to add to the sensory experience. If you feel tension or pain in your head or body while doing this, try breathing deeply into those areas, and then resume the visualization.

Do this for 5 minutes every morning this week with the goal of doing this practice for 30 minutes every day. And if you stick with this practice beyond the 6 weeks I guarantee you, your life will start to shift in ways that you can't even imagine.

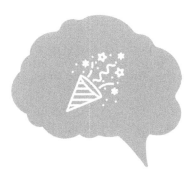

Celebrate!

CONGRATULATIONS! YOU DID IT! You have now completed your first 6-Week BrainSAVE! Plan to heal your brain from concussions, brain injuries and trauma.

I know it's not easy to dive in and make changes to your diet, take supplements every day, change your lifestyle and practice visualization. But I have a feeling that if you were 100% committed to this plan and followed through with all the recommendations that you are already feeling better. And that you now have a glimmer of hope that healing your brain is totally possible and within your reach.

I acknowledge you.

And even if you didn't do everything 100% that's okay, especially if this is your first time learning about all these cutting-edge approaches to concussion care. You can always go back and redo the 6 weeks, or the parts that you feel you need to put more energy into.

But my hope for you is that you begin to incorporate the recommendations into your everyday life so they become second nature to you, as they have for me and my patients.

And if you did do it 100% but aren't feeling any different, go back to chapter 12 and review the 12 Biggest Obstacles to Healing from Post-Concussion Syndrome, complete the self-assessment quiz, and take the recommended actions based on your score.

Reflect and Integrate

Either way, now would be a good time for you to reflect upon everything you've learned.

To conclude your 6-Week BrainSAVE! Plan, I'd like you to write down 10 things that you want to acknowledge yourself for, that you did or learned or obstacles that you were able to overcome during your 6-week plan. Anything that you'd like to acknowledge, no matter how big or small.

It's so easy to forget the many wonderful things that we're actually accomplishing every single day that move us closer to where we want to be in life, when we don't set aside some special time to reflect on it all.

So go ahead and do that now. Your brain will thank you for it.

Acknowledgements

1. _____
2. _____
3. _____
4. _____
5. _____
6. _____
7. _____
8. _____
9. _____
10. _____

Final Word

SOMETIMES IT'S IN OUR DARKEST HOURS that we are finally able to see the true light of our being. I can tell you that all the pain, suffering, sadness, loneliness and despair that I've experienced have all been invaluable teachers to me. They have changed the way I view myself, the world and others. Because on the other side of that pain and suffering was deep and profound strength, resiliency and healing.

We all have moments in all our journeys that seem hopeless, scary, lonely, frustrating— so it's what we do next that matters.

So I urge you— take the next step. Become part of the movement to transform healthcare and share your BrainSAVE! story of hope and healing with everyone you meet. Because just like my story, Karen's story and the countless other patients who have healed from their concussions– your story too can serve as a powerful source of inspiration for the millions of people around the world suffering from Post-Concussion Syndrome.

I'd like to leave you with one of my favorite poems ever. Reading it has brought great comfort to me in times of intense pain and suffering. I hope it will do the same for you.

> This being human is a guest house.
> Every morning a new arrival.
> A joy, a depression, a meanness,
> some momentary awareness comes
> as an unexpected visitor.
> Welcome and entertain them all!
> Even if they are a crowd of sorrows,
> who violently sweep your house
> empty of its furniture,
> still, treat each guest honorably.
> He may be clearing you out
> for some new delight.

–RUMI

Much hope, love and strength to you on your journey.

Dr. Titus Chiu

Functional Neurologist

www.DrTitusChiu.com

May 2018

Acknowledgments

EVER SINCE I WAS A LITTLE KID, it had always been a dream of mine to write a book. And so I feel so grateful to all the people in my life that have made this dream a reality. Obviously, from that first moment of inspiration up till now, I've encountered thousands of people that have inspired, moved, touched, and challenged me along the way. I wish I could name all of you here but that would fill pages upon pages so I'll keep this short and sweet and speak from the heart– as my grandfather had taught me to do.

I am deeply grateful to all my patients who have entrusted me with their health, and who have committed to my care. In doing so, you have all showed me what was possible with healing and the brain. You teach me every single day– in ways no textbook or classroom ever could.

To Dr. Ted Carrick, the Father of Functional Neurology. Words cannot describe the impact that you've had on my life and career (I'm sure you could very swiftly localize the longitudinal level of the lesion, but we'll save that for my next book lol). And to Dr. Jeffery Bland, the Father of Functional Medicine. It's to both of you– giants, visionaries and pioneers– that I owe much of my new ways of seeing that has helped me help thousands of patients, and allowed me to synthesize my own unique way of seeing.

Deepest gratitude goes out to all my friends and professorial colleagues in the amazing world of Functional Neurology. To you who are always pushing the envelope of what is possible with healing and the brain– Dr. Datis Kharrazian, Dr. Sam Yanuck, Dr. Glen Zielinski, Dr. Sergio Azzolino, Dr. Fili Talamantez, Dr. Robert Melillo, Dr. Brandon Brock, Dr. Marc Ellis, and Dr. Jeremy Schmoe– you guys ROCK.

And to all the countless students and doctors that I had the pleasure of teaching over the years– it was through your questions and enthusiasm and thirst for knowledge that challenged me to become a better teacher and educator. I thank you from the bottom of both my left and right prefrontal lobes.

To all my heroes and colleagues in the world of Functional Medicine– thank you for turning the tide of chronic disease and for shifting the paradigm of medicine. To Dr. David Perlmutter for his beautiful work bringing my two favorite worlds of neurology and Functional

Medicine together in such a brilliant and accessible way. To Dr. Mark Hyman for writing the Ultramind Solution, and for making Broken Brain–the ground-breaking documentary that will change the way the world sees brain disorders forever. To Dr. Kristi Hughes for being such a supportive friend and inspiration to me as an educator. And to my friends Dhru, Kaya, and Anthony for coming from such a deep, generous, and abundant place of being– you are such shining examples of truly living life from your core values.

To JJ Virgin and Karl Krummenacher for bringing together such an amazing community of movers and shakers– all on a global mission to transform health and wellness. And to Dr. Jolene Brighten for introducing me to such an extraordinary community.

To the one and only Mickey and Noah Trescott, Angie Alt, Bobby Chang and Yrmis Barroeta for inviting me into your amazing community, and for your help in getting my message out to the world in a big way– you guys are the best.

To my team at KOBA, for holding down the fort and making sure patients are taken care of while I'm out in the world speaking, teaching and writing– I appreciate you.

To my brother Dr. Timothy Chiu, for saving my life and introducing me to the wonderful world of chiropractic and natural medicine. And my sister-in-law Kelly for being such an amazing, encouraging friend– and for raising two loving kids, my adorable nephew and niece, Timmy and Bella. You all bring so much joy to my life.

To my parents for always being there for me, through thick and thin– and for giving me the physical, emotional and spiritual resources for turning my dream into a reality.

To my mother and father in-law, Mehri and Jamshid, for always loving, caring for, and supporting me as if I was your own.

To Koba for being the sweetest and most enlightened being I've ever had the pleasure to snuggle with.

And finally, to my wife, Dr. Natasha Fallahi, for all your love and support and the countless hours you waited patiently as I completed this manuscript. I've never seen a softer, bolder, more creative soul than I have in you.

BRAIN-BOOSTING RESOURCES

Dr. Titus Chiu

The Modern Brain Blog

The Modern Brain blog is written by Dr. Titus Chiu, a leader in the emerging field of Functional Neurology. 100% chock-full of quick and juicy tips to keep your mind happy, vibrant and strong.

    www.DrTitusChiu.com/articles

Modern Brain Integrative Neurology Center

Root Cause Neurology. Beautiful, state-of-the-art integrative neurology center. Innovative, natural, cutting-edge treatments in a warm and welcoming family environment. Whether you're suffering from Post-Concussion Syndrome, chronic migraines, vertigo, anxiety, depression, autoimmunity, cognitive decline, early Alzheimers or other chronic neurological symptoms, we offer a full suite of Modern Brain Treatment Programs to take your brain health to the next level.

    www.TheModernBrain.com

5-Day BrainSAVE! Recovery Program for Concussion

Application for 5-Day BrainSAVE! Recovery Program with Dr. Titus Chiu and his Modern Brain care team

    www.bit.ly/brainsaveapplication

Comprehensive Modern BrainEVAL

Advanced Functional Neurological Evaluation with Dr. Titus Chiu

    www.DrTitusChiu.com/modernbraineval

Follow Dr. Titus Chiu on Facebook

www.facebook.com/DrTitusChiu

Follow Dr. Titus Chiu on instagram

www.instagram.com/DrTitusChiu

Healing Resources:

The following Healing Resources contain links to products and services that we have researched and curated over the course of many years. We firmly believe in, personally use, and recommend these to all of our patients, family and friends. If you purchase any product or service with these links we do receive a percentage of your purchase. Not only do we think our recommendations will bring great value to your life– it will also help support our ongoing mission to transform healthcare for the 1 BILLION people around the world suffering from brain and mental disorders. Thanks for your support!

BrainSAVE! Supplements

Highest quality, Dr. Chiu curated and approved brain-boosting supplements:

www.bit.ly/brainsavesupps

Real Plans

Creative recipe and menu planning app:

www.bit.ly/realplansDTC

Sunlighten Infrared Saunas

For brain health, detoxification, anti-aging and weight loss

www.bit.ly/sunlightenKOBA

Computer filter

https://justgetflux.com

Functional Medicine and Neurology Practitioner Referrals:

Finding the right doctor or practitioner who can get to the root cause for your symptoms, is current with the latest research, who understands the ins and outs of your unique situation, and who you trust and resonate with is no simple task.

Here is a list of organizations that can help you find a practitioner trained in the different cutting-edge treatments that I use in my practice. The experience, background, training and skills of each person will differ from practitioner to practitioner, so it's up to you to do your homework in finding the best practitioner for your unique neurological needs.

Functional Medicine

The Institute for Functional Medicine

www.ifm.org

Functional Neurology

American Chiropractic Neurology Board

www.acnb.org

Functional Nutrition and Health Coaching

Functional Medicine Coaching Academy

www.functionalmedicinecoaching.org

NOTES

[1] Tagge CA, Fisher AM, Minaeva OV, et al. Concussion, microvascular injury, and early tauopathy in young athletes after impact head injury and an impact concussion mouse model. *Brain*. 2018;141(2):422-458. doi:10.1093/brain/awx350.

2 Traumatic Brain Injury & Concussion. Centers for Disease Control and Prevention. https://www.cdc.gov/traumaticbraininjury/get_the_facts.html. Published April 27, 2017. Accessed May 1, 2018.

[3] Schwarzbold M, Diaz A, Martins ET, et al. Psychiatric disorders and traumatic brain injury. *Neuropsychiatric Disease and Treatment*. 2008;4(4):797-816.

[4] Barnes DE, Byers AL, Gardner RC, Seal KH, Boscardin WJ, Yaffe K. Association of Mild Traumatic Brain Injury With and Without Loss of Consciousness With Dementia in US Military Veterans. *JAMA Neurol*. Published online May 07, 2018. doi:10.1001/jamaneurol.2018.0815

[5] Lye TC & Shores EA. Traumatic brain injury as a risk factor for Alzheimer's disease: a review. *Neuropsychol Rev*. 2000 Jun;10(2):115-29.

[6] Gardner Raquel C., Byers Amy L., Barnes Deborah E., Li Yixia, Boscardin John, Yaffe Kristine. Mild TBI and risk of Parkinson disease. *Neurology*. Apr 2018, 10.1212/WNL.0000000000005522; DOI: 10.1212/WNL.0000000000005522

[7] Jiunn-Horng Kang & Herng-Ching Lin. Increased risk of multiple sclerosis after traumatic brain injury: a nationwide population-based study. *Journal of Neurotrauma*. 2012 Jan 1;29(1):90-5.

[8] Traumatic Brain Injury & Concussion. Centers for Disease Control and Prevention. https://www.cdc.gov/traumaticbraininjury/get_the_facts.html. Published April 27, 2017. Accessed May 1, 2018.

[9] Bansal V, Costantini T, Kroll L, et al. Traumatic Brain Injury and Intestinal Dysfunction: Uncovering the Neuro-Enteric Axis. *Journal of Neurotrauma*. 2009;26(8):1353-1359. doi:10.1089/neu.2008.0858.

[10] Fasano, A. Leaky gut and autoimmune diseases. *Clinical Reviews in Allergy and Immunology*. (2012) 42: 71. https://doi.org/10.1007/s12016-011-8291-x

[11] Blaylock RL, Maroon J. Immunoexcitotoxicity as a central mechanism in chronic traumatic encephalopathy—A unifying hypothesis. *Surgical Neurology International*. 2011;2:107. doi:10.4103/2152-7806.83391.

[12] Fuchs, Eberhard & Flugge, Gabriele. (2014). Adult Neuroplasticity: More Than 40 Years of Research. *Neural plasticity*. 2014. 541870. 10.1155/2014/541870.

[13] Merzenich, Michael M, Van Vleet, Thomas M, & Nahum, Mor. Brain plasticity-based therapeutics. *Front Hum. Neurosci.* 27 Jun 2014; https://doi.org/10.3389/fnhum.2014.00385.

[14] Shaffer J. Neuroplasticity and Clinical Practice: Building Brain Power for Health. *Frontiers in Psychology*. 2016;7:1118. doi:10.3389/fpsyg.2016.01118.

[15] Cramer SC, Sur M, Dobkin BH, et al. Harnessing neuroplasticity for clinical applications. *Brain*. 2011;134(6):1591-1609. doi:10.1093/brain/awr039.

[16] Phillips C. Lifestyle Modulators of Neuroplasticity: How Physical Activity, Mental Engagement, and Diet Promote Cognitive Health during Aging. *Neural Plasticity*. 2017;2017:3589271. doi:10.1155/2017/3589271.

[17] May, Arne. Experience-dependent structural plasticity in the adult human brain. *Trends in Cognitive Sciences*. 15(10): 475-482.

[18] Gaser, Christian & Schlaug, Gottfried. Gray Matter Differences between Musicians and Nonmusicians. *Annals of the New York Academy of Sciences*. 24 Jan 2006; 999(1). doi.org/10.1196/annals.1284.062

[19] Kleim JA & Jones TA. Principles of experience-dependent neural plasticity: implications for rehabilitation after brain damage. *J Speech Lang Hear Res*. 2008 Feb;51(1):S225-39. doi: 10.1044/1092-4388(2008/018).

[20] Carrick FR, Clark JF, Pagnacco G, et al. Head–Eye Vestibular Motion Therapy Affects the Mental and Physical Health of Severe Chronic Postconcussion Patients. *Frontiers in Neurology*. 2017;8:414. doi:10.3389/fneur.2017.00414.

[21] Huang, Ying-Ying & Gupta, Asheesh & Vecchio, Daniela & J Bil de Arce, Vida & Huang, Shih-Fong & Xuan, Weijun & Hamblin, Michael. (2012). Transcranial low level laser (light) therapy for traumatic brain injury. *Journal of biophotonics*. 5. 10.1002/jbio.201200077.

[22] K.J. Brown, V. Jewells, H. Herfarth, & M. Castillo. White Matter Lesions Suggestive of Amyotrophic Lateral Sclerosis Attributed to Celiac Disease. *American Journal of Neuroradiology*. May 2010, 31 (5) 880-881; DOI: 10.3174/ajnr.A1826

[23] Masafumi Ihara, Fumi Makino, Hideyuki Sawada, Takahiro Mezaki, Kotaro Mizutani, Hiroshi Nakase, Makoto Matsui, Hidekazu Tomimoto, Shun Shimohama, Gluten Sensitivity in Japanese Patients with Adultonset Cerebellar Ataxia. *Internal Medicine*. Released March 01, 2006, Online ISSN 1349-7235, Print ISSN 0918-2918, https://doi.org/10.2169/internalmedicine.45.1351.

[24] Hadjivassiliou M, Grünewald RA, Davies-Jones GAB Gluten sensitivity as a neurological illness. *Journal of Neurology, Neurosurgery & Psychiatry.* 2002;72:560-563.

[25] Gallaway, Michael, Scheiman, Mitchell, & Mitchell, G. Lynn. Vision Therapy for Post-Concussion Vision Disorders. *Optometry and Vision Science.* Jan 2017;94(1):68-73. doi: 10.1097/OPX.0000000000000935

[26] Gustavo Rocha Peixoto dos Santos João, Silva Paiva Wellingson, and Jacobsen Teixeira Manoel. Transcranial light-emitting diode therapy for neuropsychological improvement after traumatic brain injury: a new perspective for diffuse axonal lesion management. *Med Devices (Auckl).* 2018;11:139-146. Published online 2018 Apr 26. doi: 10.2147/MDER.S155356

[27] Hamblin Michael R. Photobiomodulation for traumatic brain injury and stroke. *Journal of Neuroscience Research.* 13 Nov 2017; 96(4). doi.org/10.1002/jnr.24190

[28] Lamb DG, Porges EC, Lewis GF, Williamson JB. Non-invasive Vagal Nerve Stimulation Effects on Hyperarousal and Autonomic State in Patients with Post-traumatic Stress Disorder and History of Mild Traumatic Brain Injury: Preliminary Evidence. *Frontiers in Medicine.* 2017;4:124. doi:10.3389/fmed.2017.00124.

[29] Gurley, James M., Hujsak, Bryan D., Kelly, Jennifer L. Vestibular rehabilitation following mild traumatic brain injury. *NeuroRehabilitation.* 2013;32(3): 519-528.

[30] Khalsa DS. Stress, Meditation, and Alzheimer's Disease Prevention: Where The Evidence Stands. Ashford JW, ed. *Journal of Alzheimer's Disease.* 2015;48(1):1-12. doi:10.3233/JAD-142766.

[31] Lulu Xie, Hongyi Kang, Qiwu Xu, Michael J. Chen, Yonghong Liao, Meenakshisundaram Thiyagarajan, John O'Donnell, Daniel J. Christensen, Charles Nicholson, Jeffrey J. Iliff, Takahiro Takano, Rashid Deane, Maiken Nedergaard. Sleep Drives Metabolite Clearance from the Adult Brain. *Science.* 18 Oct 2013 : 373-377

[32] Kirste, Imke & Nicola, Zeina & Kronenberg, Golo & Walker, Tara & Liu, Robert & Kempermann, Gerd. (2013). Is silence golden? Effects of auditory stimuli and their absence on adult hippocampal neurogenesis. *Brain structure & function.* 10.1007/s00429-013-0679-3.

[33] Body Burden: The Pollution in Newborns. *Environmental Working Group.* 14 July 2005. https://www.ewg.org/research/body-burden-pollution-new-borns#.Wv1_GyPMzVp

About the Author

Dr. Titus Chiu is a #1 bestselling author, award-winning international speaker, and Functional Neurologist who is on a mission to transform the face of healthcare for the 1 billion people around the world struggling with brain and mental disorders.

Through his professional and personal experiences as a professor, doctor, and concussion survivor, Dr. Chiu has treated thousands of patients and trained thousands of doctors and healthcare professionals from around the world.

He is the creator of Root Cause Neurology, a holistic, cutting-edge approach to brain health that blends ancient Eastern wisdom practices with the latest breakthroughs in neurology, nutrition and genomic medicine.

Dr. Chiu has a deep passion for teaching and had the honor to present at the 2017 Institute for Functional Medicine's Annual International Conference on the Brain. He was also featured on Dr. Mark Hyman's groundbreaking documentary Broken Brain.

Dr. Chiu is the co-founder and clinical director of KOBA family wellness, a Functional Medicine center located in Berkeley, California that specializes in helping people struggling with chronic brain and autoimmune conditions get well and stay well.

He lives in Berkeley, California with his wife and their Rhodesian Ridgeback, Koba.

Made in the USA
Middletown, DE
19 December 2018